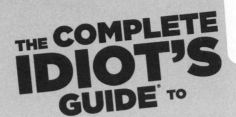

# Eating Paleo

by Neely Quinn, ICNT, CLT, and Jason Glaspey

**ALPHA**

A member of Penguin Group (USA) Inc.

*This book is dedicated to all the archaeologists, anthropologists, and other researchers, without whom we wouldn't have this precious, life-changing information.*

## ALPHA BOOKS

Published by the Penguin Group

Penguin Group (USA) Inc., 375 Hudson Street, New York, New York 10014, USA • Penguin Group (Canada), 90 Eglinton Avenue East, Suite 700, Toronto, Ontario M4P 2Y3, Canada (a division of Pearson Penguin Canada Inc.) • Penguin Books Ltd., 80 Strand, London WC2R 0RL, England • Penguin Ireland, 25 St. Stephen's Green, Dublin 2, Ireland (a division of Penguin Books Ltd.) • Penguin Group (Australia), 250 Camberwell Road, Camberwell, Victoria 3124, Australia (a division of Pearson Australia Group Pty. Ltd.) • Penguin Books India Pvt. Ltd., 11 Community Centre, Panchsheel Park, New Delhi—110 017, India • Penguin Group (NZ), 67 Apollo Drive, Rosedale, North Shore, Auckland 1311, New Zealand (a division of Pearson New Zealand Ltd.) • Penguin Books (South Africa) (Pty.) Ltd., 24 Sturdee Avenue, Rosebank, Johannesburg 2196, South Africa • Penguin Books Ltd., Registered Offices: 80 Strand, London WC2R 0RL, England

## Copyright © 2012 by Neely Quinn and Jason Glaspey

THE COMPLETE IDIOT'S GUIDE TO and Design are registered trademarks of Penguin Group (USA) Inc.

International Standard Book Number: 978-1-61564-149-9
Library of Congress Catalog Card Number: 2011938639

17  16       14  13  12  11

Interpretation of the printing code: The rightmost number of the first series of numbers is the year of the book's printing; the rightmost number of the second series of numbers is the number of the book's printing. For example, a printing code of 12-1 shows that the first printing occurred in 2012.

*Printed in the United States of America*

**Note:** This publication contains the opinions and ideas of its authors. It is intended to provide helpful and informative material on the subject matter covered. It is sold with the understanding that the authors and publisher are not engaged in rendering professional services in the book. If the reader requires personal assistance or advice, a competent professional should be consulted.

The authors and publisher specifically disclaim any responsibility for any liability, loss, or risk, personal or otherwise, which is incurred as a consequence, directly or indirectly, of the use and application of any of the contents of this book.

Most Alpha books are available at special quantity discounts for bulk purchases for sales promotions, premiums, fund-raising, or educational use. Special books, or book excerpts, can also be created to fit specific needs. For details, write: Special Markets, Alpha Books, 375 Hudson Street, New York, NY 10014.

**Publisher:** *Marie Butler-Knight*
**Associate Publisher:** *Mike Sanders*
**Executive Managing Editor:** *Billy Fields*
**Senior Acquisitions Editor:** *Brook Farling*
**Development Editor:** *Lynn Northrup*
**Senior Production Editor:** *Kayla Dugger*

**Copy Editor:** *Cate Schwenk*
**Cover Designer:** *William Thomas*
**Book Designers:** *William Thomas, Rebecca Batchelor*
**Indexer:** *Celia McCoy*
**Layout:** *Ayanna Lacey*
**Senior Proofreader:** *Laura Caddell*

# Contents

## Appendixes

# Foreword

I've written a couple of forewords for other authors in the Primal/Paleo/ancestral health realm, and every time I tell people (who don't really get this whole Primal thing) what I'm about to do, someone invariably asks, "But aren't they your competition?"

That's a silly way to think about it, but I understand where they're coming from. A lot of folks in other industries guard secrets very closely, because it's easy to see your peers as vying for your slice of the pie. Because, well, the pie is usually a lot smaller, and grabbing your slice might require someone else not getting one. Not here. Nope—the Primal/Paleo pie is a big, grain-free one that's growing every day with plenty of slices to go around for everyone. As long as you have something to offer, some new perspective, angle, or way of approaching the problem of evolutionary health, nutrition, and fitness, there is an audience of people who desperately need it.

I mean, just look at the people around you. Diabetes, obesity, arthritis, depression, and other chronic diseases are everywhere. People work long hours, sleep very little, sit all day, and self-medicate with TV and computer time. Kids don't really play outside anymore, instead choosing to stay indoors glued to the screen. So there's a definite need for more avenues into the evolutionary health movement, and that need is getting bigger every day.

The funny thing is that, although eating in accordance with our ancestors should be simple, intuitive, and the totally natural thing to do, that doesn't mean some people couldn't use a little help getting started. We are, after all, what MovNat creator Erwan Le Corre calls "zoo humans"—animals who manage to maintain a lifestyle that is diametrically opposed to their fundamental natures. We've forgotten the basics, and we've lost the intuitive connection to our own bodies, appetites, and health. It's a sick slide down a slippery slope and it needs to stop.

*The Complete Idiot's Guide to Eating Paleo* is the perfect crash course for regaining that essential connection. It's direct, practical, and utilitarian, with the perfect amount of style and personality provided by authors Neely and Jason. They break down this whole "regaining health and wellness through nutrition while bypassing the traditional medical community" thing—a fairly daunting responsibility for one to assume, don't you think?—into bite-sized, easily digestible pieces to make it doable. They remove the guesswork so you can focus on feeling better.

Whatever you call it—Primal, Paleo, caveman, ancestral, stone-age—it's about making eating, exercising, sleeping, and simply staying healthy as simple as possible. At least that's the idea, right? The big problem is that getting to the point where this stuff becomes second nature requires surviving a rough transition where all your previously held beliefs about, well, everything are heavily and mercilessly scrutinized. It can leave a person feeling pretty unsettled and unsure.

*The Complete Idiot's Guide to Eating Paleo* is the antidote to that transition. Read it, use it, and prepare for a healthy new life.

Mark Sisson, author of *The Primal Blueprint*

# Introduction

Maybe you've seen family or friends lose weight on the Paleolithic diet. Or maybe it's just that it's popping up all over the internet and magazines, and you want to know what the heck this diet is all about. Well, you've picked up the right book because the following pages spell out this anti-inflammatory diet simply and thoroughly. We not only give you good, scientific reasons for eating Paleo, but we also provide you with the recipes, meal plans, and the know-how to make it work with your lifestyle immediately.

The Paleolithic diet goes against a lot of conventional wisdom. Fat is bad, meat is bad, and whole grains are good: those are all things we've been told for years as truths. This book will dispel those myths and others and help you put an end to weight gain and perhaps even reverse diabetes and heart disease. You can get those ripped muscles, painless joints, and the perfect skin you've always wanted, just by changing a few things about your diet. In this book, you learn the *real* basics of good nutrition—the kind of nutrition that we, and our Paleolithic ancestors, were born to thrive on.

## How This Book Is Organized

We've broken this book up into four parts to help make it easily digestible and simple to follow. Each part provides you with different information to help guide you through the background, implementation, cooking, and meal planning of the Paleolithic diet.

**Part 1, All About Paleo,** navigates the history behind the diet and the scientific affirmations for eating and living Paleo. You find out what our primitive ancestors ate and why they didn't suffer from diabetes, heart disease, obesity, and other modern afflictions. We tell you exactly what foods are Paleo and which aren't, and we even discuss the debatable Paleo foods. You find out how much protein, fat, and carbohydrates you should optimally be eating, and we dispel some myths about higher protein and fat diets. Finally, you get to see some modern research that shows that this diet really works.

**Part 2, Implementing Paleo,** is all about making the simple diet of our Paleolithic ancestors work for us in our modern world. Whether you're an athlete, a mother of three, or a frequent traveler, this diet can work for you. You find tips for cleaning out your kitchen, stocking it up right, and making the diet sustainable. You also find out about the less common ingredients in the diet and how to use them properly.

**Part 3, Paleo-Perfect Recipes,** introduces you to some delicious, satisfying Paleo recipes! You need to know what to eat on this diet, so we've provided you with a boatload of mouthwatering breakfasts, snacks and salads, appetizers and sides, dinners, and desserts. You should be able to thoroughly impress, and maybe even convert, your friends and family with these dishes. This part of the book gives you the tools you need to really incorporate this diet into your life for good. Unlike other diets, this food is what we evolved eating, so it's incredibly satisfying.

**Part 4, Meal Planning,** brings the book full circle with a meal plan. Even with the recipes and all the other important information in the book, you may not have the time or patience to put it into practice. The meal plan in this part provides you with 4 weeks of menus and grocery shopping lists, using the recipes in the book as the backbone. You get some practical tips on how to effectively use and alter the meal plan if you need to, as well as information on counting calories. Also in this part, you find out what to expect in the first month and how to avoid common beginner mistakes.

We also include five helpful appendixes: a glossary of terms we use throughout the book; resources for foods and other products, as well as further reading and other good-to-know stuff; grocery shopping lists for the meal plan; and some very enlightening nutritional information on the major macronutrients as well as how the Paleolithic diet stacks up against the traditional Western diet.

## Extras

As you read through the book, you will notice bonus sidebars that contain definitions, tips, warnings, and miscellaneous information to help you better understand the subject matter.

**DEFINITION**

These sidebars provide you with definitions that are relevant to the topic at hand.

**PALEO COMPASS**

Check these sidebars for tips to stay on track, interesting Paleo facts and explanations of Paleo concepts, and miscellaneous related information.

**DAMAGE CONTROL**

These sidebars contain cautions you should keep in mind when it comes to the Paleo lifestyle.

**NUTRITION FACT**

These sidebars are full of practical nutritional Information that might just surprise you.

## Acknowledgments

First of all, thank you to all the anthropologists, archaeologists, nutrition researchers, philosophers, bloggers, and authors out there who've paved the way for the Paleo movement.

Our deepest gratitude is owed to Molly Pearl Owen and the Paleo Plan Team for their hard work on the recipes in this book. Molly's excellent taste and attention to detail are evident in every one of the dishes presented in this book.

We would like to thank our subscribers at Paleo Plan. Their questions about the diet provided great insight into the information that was difficult to understand and needed extra focus. Also, their suggestions for the recipes were crucial in the final editing process.

Special thanks go to Marilyn Allen of the Allen O'Shea Literary Agency, for having faith in us to do this book justice. Also to Brook Farling, acquisitions editor at Alpha Books, for guiding the process from beginning to end with gentleness and an open mind.

Neely would like to thank her first nutritional anthropology teacher, Paul Bergner, who opened her eyes to the hunter-gatherer way. Neely thanks her co-author, Jason Glaspey, for his excellent feedback and partnership through this process. And of course, much love and gratitude go to Neely's boyfriend, Seth, for his patience and understanding during the writing process; and to her family and friends for their continued support and encouragement.

Jason would like to offer his sincere appreciation to Scott Hagnas of CrossFit Portland, for planting the original seeds of eating Paleo and what that really meant. To Mike Pacchione, Meg Valas, and Doug Gould, for helping to make sense of hundreds of recipes and gathering facts and nutrition information through tireless data entry. To the Portland Incubator Experiment, where Paleo Plan was born, and where much of this book was put together. And to Holly, his lovely wife, who graciously puts up with a lot.

## Special Thanks to the Technical Reviewer

*The Complete Idiot's Guide to Eating Paleo* was reviewed by an expert who double-checked the accuracy of what you learn here. She helped ensure that this book gives you everything you need to know about the Paleolithic diet, and that the recipes are delicious and undoubtedly Paleo. Special thanks are extended to Karen Rylander.

Karen Rylander is a trained personal chef specializing in Paleo-inspired meals and snacks. She has a B.A. in Anthropology from University of Colorado Boulder and completed her certification as a Holistic Nutrition Consultant in December 2011. Karen has been eating Paleo for over 2 years.

## Trademarks

All terms mentioned in this book that are known to be or are suspected of being trademarks or service marks have been appropriately capitalized. Alpha Books and Penguin Group (USA) Inc. cannot attest to the accuracy of this information. Use of a term in this book should not be regarded as affecting the validity of any trademark or service mark.

# All About Paleo

The Paleolithic diet is time tested and science approved. It turns out that eating a primitive diet like our Paleolithic ancestors did (with a modern twist) could potentially change your life and health forever. Grains, dairy, refined sugar, vegetable oils, and unnecessary additives are all foods that our Paleolithic ancestors didn't eat, and the lack of them may have led to their excellent health.

When you focus on eating meat, fish, eggs, vegetables, fruit, and some nuts and seeds, you'll find you lose weight, have better digestion, more stable moods, better athletic performance, beautiful skin, and plenty of nutrients.

The Paleolithic diet is often thought to be a low-carb high-protein diet, but it doesn't have to be. While eating a lower carbohydrate diet will definitely help you lose weight, the diet can be whatever you need it to be; as long as you stay away from non-Paleo foods, you're all good.

# Paleo 101

**In This Chapter**

- What is the Paleolithic diet?
- Why this way of eating works
- The foods our Paleolithic ancestors ate
- The problems with agricultural foods

The Paleolithic diet (also known as the caveman diet, Stone Age diet, or hunter-gatherer diet) aims to mimic what our Paleolithic ancestors ate: meat, fish, eggs, vegetables, fruits, nuts, and seeds. It's a straightforward and satisfying way to lose weight and reclaim your health.

The Paleolithic diet is time tested like no other diet: 2.5 million years, in fact. In other words, it's been around for all of human (or hominid) life on Earth. This way of eating proves that not all things old are outdated. It's an ancient way of eating, but modern research shows that it works. You might think that people long ago lived short, brutal lives, wherein they didn't live long enough to even develop chronic diseases of today. But there's actually a lot of evidence that many of them lived to ripe old ages—into their 60s, 70s, and beyond, but free of modern maladies like diabetes, obesity, cancer, and heart disease. In fact, it seems that our Paleolithic ancestors and modern hunter-gatherer groups were and are the muscular, energetic, healthy people we want to be.

The Paleolithic era began about 2.5 million years ago, marked by the use of the first stone tools. It ended about 10,000 years ago, or 330 generations ago, with the start of the Neolithic era, marked by the advent of agriculture and animal domestication.

During the Paleolithic era, people didn't have grocery stores, food processing plants, dairies, or even crops of food. Before people settled down and started farming, everyone lived and thrived on foods they could hunt, scavenge, or forage. The modern Western diet is a huge departure from that, 70 percent of which is comprised of agricultural foods like grains, legumes (beans), dairy, refined sugars, and vegetable oils.

This chapter gives you an overview of what ancient and modern hunter-gatherers ate and didn't eat, and how that can translate into our modern world.

# Not Just a Diet

Although we use the word "diet" in this book a lot, we don't mean it in the way you're used to hearing it. "Diet" usually refers to something you go on, which implies that you'll eventually go *off* of it once you reach your goal weight or your health goals. The difference between fad diets and this one is that Paleo is meant to be a lifestyle— not just a passing phase.

You will probably reach those weight and health goals eating Paleo, but if you go back to your old ways of eating immediately afterward, you'll eventually just end up back where you were. Luckily for you, it's a sustainable diet, so you'll be able to stick with it for life.

# Eating the Paleo Way

This diet is simple and doable. There's no need to starve yourself, count points, weigh food, or tediously keep track of calories or carbohydrates. If you just switch out the foods in your kitchen with those our hunter-gatherer ancestors ate, you will be well on your way to sustainable health (and that body you've always wanted).

Hunter-gatherers went where there was abundant and wild food to be found. To eat Paleo, we're not saying you need to give up your earthly belongings and go live in the woods, hunting elk and picking berries; you can hunt and gather everything you need at your local grocery store to successfully mimic our ancestors.

Why should you change your whole diet? Maybe you feel okay most days and don't think you need a complete diet overhaul. Unfortunately, sometimes people don't feel the effects of chronic illnesses developing until it's too late. You may not feel inflammation in your arteries, but that doesn't mean you won't suffer a heart attack someday.

Plus, sometimes people don't even notice life-long symptoms until they change their diet and discover how much better they can feel. You might think that feeling bloated after every meal, feeling fatigued every afternoon, and gaining weight as you get older are just normal parts of life, but they're not. You'll find a comprehensive explanation of the benefits of the diet in Chapter 2, but here are some of the positive changes you might see if you switch to eating Paleo:

- Weight loss and muscle gain

- Stable blood sugar

- More sustained energy throughout the day

- Better digestion—less burping, heartburn, constipation, diarrhea, and bloating

- Less sinus congestion

- Fewer allergy symptoms

- More stable moods

- Healthier skin

- Better reproductive health

- Healthier joints—less pain

- Improved athletic performance

- Fewer food cravings

# What Our Ancestors Ate

So what exactly *did* our Paleolithic ancestors eat, since grains, *legumes*, dairy, sugar, and vegetable oils make up the bulk of a modern diet? How do you go about mimicking them? The truth is that all hunter-gatherer diets shared some commonalities, but they were sometimes quite different from each other. It all depended on where they were living and what was available to them.

**DEFINITION**

A **legume** is a plant in the family *Fabaceae,* and includes pinto and black beans, lentils, soy, and peanuts.

Dr. Loren Cordain, one of the fathers of the Paleolithic diet and author of *The Paleo Diet* (see Appendix B), collaborated on a study published in the *Journal of the American Nutraceutical Association* in 2002, in which the diets of 229 primitive societies were analyzed. The study found that on average, 25 to 35 percent of their diet was made up of plant foods and 56 to 65 percent was animal foods. However, that's just an average. There's not one diet that is *the* Paleolithic diet, but there are definitely guidelines we can glean from the successful diets of hunter-gatherers.

Here are the diets of a handful of hunter-gatherer groups from Paleolithic times and today:

- Sometime around 2 million years ago in Ethiopia, a predecessor to modern humans known as *Australopithecus garhi* was eating catfish as well as the meat, tongues, and fatty marrow out of the bones of horses and antelopes.

- Researchers found remains of wild plants, boars, gazelles, deer, and tortoises that were cooked over an open fire by a group of Mousterian people living in northern Israel 200,000 years ago.

- Around 10,000 years ago, hunter-gatherers in the Rocky Mountains of Colorado were eating camel, mammoth, bison, sloth, mountain sheep, beaver, pronghorn antelope, elk, mule deer, horse, llama, and large members of the dog family. They were also gathering foods like sunflower seeds, berries, roots, bulbs, and leaves from various plants.

- In the early 1900s, the Inuit of Alaska ate salmon, salmon eggs, seals, walrus, other fish, and seal oil. The fish was often dipped in seal oil before being dried. From the land, they hunted caribou, moose, reindeer, birds, and other game. In the summer, they gathered nuts, kelp, berries, and flower blossoms and sorrel preserved in seal oil. They also prized the organs they harvested from larger sea animals, like whale skin and seal livers.

**PALEO COMPASS**

Depending on what they could store from their summer foraging, the Inuit people sometimes ate a diet of 100 percent animal foods for six to nine months of the year. In 1928, in an attempt to show the medical community that the Inuit diet was perfectly healthy, an Arctic explorer named Vilhjalmur Stefansson ate only muscle and organ meats for an entire year. At the end of his year-long, animal-only diet, he was found by the medical community to be perfectly healthy, astounding his naysayers.

- Today the primitive Kitavans of the Trobriand Islands in Papua New Guinea's archipelago eat a combination of root vegetables (yam, sweet potato, taro, and tapioca), fruit (banana, papaya, pineapple, mango, guava, watermelon, and pumpkin), vegetables, fish, and coconuts.

As you can see, all the primitive diets differ from each other in ways, but they're all similar in that they consisted of wild animal products and wild plant matter. Some, like the modern-day Kitavans, eat relatively few animal foods, while others ate mostly animal products, especially at certain times of the year. There are even some very successful primal societies, like the Masaai in Africa, who have domesticated cattle and made raw milk products a staple of their diet. None of them, however, regularly ate grains, legumes, refined sugars, or refined vegetable oils.

But were they healthy? There have been countless observations of hunter-gatherer societies in the past 300 years, as well as findings from the frozen remains of ancient people. The most notable and consistent finding among hunter-gatherer societies is the absence of both modern foods and modern, chronic diseases. In addition to that, recent studies have shown that eating a Paleolithic diet like theirs is highly effective with weight loss, and can help reverse and prevent diabetes and heart disease.

# Where We Went Wrong

For unknown reasons about 10,000 years ago, nomadic hunting and gathering began to give way to settling in one place, raising crops, and keeping domesticated animals. One theory is that drought and a lack of animal prey drove people to subsist on plant foods. The first crops were grains and legumes, likely harvested for their relatively high protein content.

Agriculture became a mainstay in society because grain and legume crops, along with domesticated animals, were readily available sources of food. They helped societies become more stable, rooted, and secure. Having a constant source of food to sustain a whole tribe of people freed up time for cultural advancements like written language, academics, and commerce.

While those crop foods helped the advancement of humanity, it's likely they also played an instrumental role in the overwhelming predominance of heart disease, digestive problems, immune disorders, diabetes, and obesity rates throughout the world. And the speed at which these previously unknown foods were adopted as staples of our diet was significant. Our genes have not had time to catch up with the changes.

There have been major health declines since agriculture took hold of humanity, including:

- Decreased average height
- Increased dental cavities and gum disease
- Increased cancer rates
- Increased osteoporosis and arthritis
- Increased body fat/decreased muscle
- Skyrocketing type 2 diabetes rates
- More heart disease
- Iron-deficient anemia
- Widespread nutrient deficiencies

**DAMAGE CONTROL**

According to a study done in 2003, it's possible that myopia, or near-sightedness, may even have something to do with eating Neolithic, high-carbohydrate foods. One study found a correlation between eating too many carbohydrates (grains, sugar, and legumes) and children developing myopia! Apparently, all those extra carbs tamper with the hormonal regulation of normal eye growth.

So what's so bad about the foods that were introduced into our diet? What is it about them that we can't tolerate? We go into much more detail about the physical effects of these foods in Chapter 2, but for now, here's an overview.

## Grains and Legumes

You'll find lists of grains and legumes in Chapter 3 if you're not sure what they are. Grains are found in foods like bread, pasta, crackers, cookies, granola, rice, and cereal. Legumes, or beans, are things like soy, black beans, and peanuts.

Some hunter-gatherer groups ate grass seeds and certain legumes, but not in the form of refined wheat flour, tofu, or corn oil. Such seeds are pretty energy inefficient to collect, thus they were never considered as staples like they are today. In their raw form, grains and legumes are toxic, and people figured that out very early on. Even when they're cooked, seeds and grains contain gluten and *antinutrients*, like certain lectins, phytic acid, and enzyme inhibitors, which are detrimental to our health. Antinutrients interfere with the absorption of nutrients, and gluten can cause intestinal damage and immune problems. There's research that links lectins and gluten with autoimmune disorders, immune responses to foods, neurological disorders, skin problems, and major intestinal diseases. There are hundreds of symptoms and illnesses that may have their roots in grain and legume intolerance.

**DEFINITION**

An **antinutrient** is a natural or synthetic compound that interferes with the absorption of nutrients. Examples include phytic acid and enzyme inhibitors in grains and the tannins in wine.

If the antinutrients weren't bad enough, we've gone and made things worse by refining grains in order to get the whitest, fluffiest baked goods possible. Refined grains are made by removing the bran and germ from whole grains. What's left is the carbohydrate-rich endosperm and very few nutrients—in other words, empty calories. Due to their lack of fiber and nutrients, refined grains cause blood sugar imbalances, which cause cravings for more refined grains and sugars; it's a vicious cycle.

When you eat foods like refined sugars and grains that are stripped of nutrients, you actually use up your own precious stores of vitamins and minerals to digest and assimilate them, instead of using the nutrients that are naturally part of whole foods.

You may be thinking there must be some mistake: you've always heard that grains are an integral part of a healthy diet. Grains are supposed to be good for us! In fact, they were the foundation of the USDA's Food Pyramid. So how could they be bad for us?

We understand that you'll probably put up a fight about cutting grains out of your diet. Our consumption of grains has dramatically increased in the United States in the last 40 years by 45 percent, constituting a whopping 24 percent of the American diet. Grains are delicious, but they may also be addictive! Opioid peptides called gliadorphins are formed during digestion of gluten grains, and it's hypothesized that they have an opioid effect on people, producing a sense of euphoria just like some drugs do. A 2005 study published in the journal *Life Sciences* found that gliadorphins can stimulate the same blissful hormone, prolactin, that opioid drugs stimulate. In fact, it's not uncommon for people to go through a withdrawal period when they first give up gluten grains, similar to what one might go through when quitting pain killers or heroin. Their addictive property alone is a decent reason to give them up.

Regardless of the potentially harmful properties of grains, the American Health Association and the American Dietetics Association continue to tout them as being healthy for us. Maybe those organizations are being influenced by grain and sugar lobbyists to keep quiet about the real detriments of bread, pasta, and corn. Or perhaps they haven't seen the research and they're just passing along outdated information with good intentions. Or maybe after so many millennia of eating grains, we've just collectively forgotten that there could be any other way.

## Refined Sugars

Although a lot of hunter-gatherers took advantage of honey and maple syrup seasonally (and some ate quite a bit of it), they didn't have refined cane sugar, high-fructose corn syrup (now marketed as corn sugar), rice syrup, corn syrup, refined maple syrup, or other refined sugars we have now.

> **PALEO COMPASS**
>
> Native American hunter-gatherers sometimes added maple syrup to pemmican, a traditional food that was made from dried buffalo meat and berries and then sealed in buffalo fat. The mixture was made into a bar and used as traveling food because it was naturally preserved for long periods of time, and it was nutrient and energy rich. Pemmican sustained Native Americans through long, winter treks and kept them free of scurvy.

Simple sugars like *glucose* and fructose are not necessarily bad for us. They're naturally found in foods like fruit and honey. However, the sugars in those foods come naturally packaged with nutrients to help digest and assimilate the sugar, and fiber to soften the blow to blood sugar levels. But when the fiber and nutrients are stripped away, like with table sugar and corn sugar, you're left with refined sugars. Added sugars make up about 16 percent of the U.S. diet, at 152 pounds of sweeteners per year per person. That's about 40 percent more than people ate as recently as the 1950s. As we all know, the statistic that has sadly followed the increased sugar consumption is the swell in obesity and diabetes rates: from 1950 to 2010, obesity in the United States increased 348 percent.

> **DEFINITION**
>
> **Glucose** is a type of carbohydrate that is a simple sugar made of carbon, oxygen, and hydrogen. It's an important energy source in living organisms, and it's a building block for many other carbohydrates.

Too much refined sugar can cause serious blood sugar imbalances. Chronically high blood sugar leads to high triglycerides and impaired cholesterol levels. It also creates high insulin levels, which can lead to insulin resistance and diabetes, and of course, obesity. Diabetes and obesity are risk factors for heart disease, which is the number one cause of death in the United States.

Sugar can also contribute to nutrient depletions, mood disorders, skin problems, intestinal inflammation, and fatigue. It promotes the growth of yeast and bacteria in your intestines and contributes to chronic inflammation. It also depletes antioxidants, weakening your immune system.

We evolved without a constant source of sugar, but when it was available, it was a hot commodity due to the fact that it's a quick source of energy. It's instinctive for us to overeat it. African pygmy people climb 100-foot trees to battle bees for their honey-filled hives, risking their lives for the stuff. Nobody blames you for wanting sugar, but what you should understand is that your desire wasn't meant to be fulfilled every time you crave it. The constant availability has drastically multiplied the rate at which we consume sugar—and its effect on our health is tremendous.

Modern hunter-gatherers (such as the Kitavans, a nonagricultural group living in Papua New Guinea) who've had blood work done have normal blood sugar levels. They also don't have impaired cholesterol or triglyceride levels, meaning heart disease is incredibly rare among them. In fact, no Kitavan—not even a 100-year-old man who was interviewed by researchers—had ever seen anyone die suddenly, as if from a heart attack or stroke. Hunter-gatherers are almost never overweight, and they often have impressive muscle tone.

## Dairy

The topic of dairy is hotly debated in the Paleo community. While it's generally accepted that grains, legumes, refined sugar, and vegetable oils are big no-no's, dairy is still on the proverbial table. Some experts believe it's a perfectly acceptable part of a Paleo lifestyle, especially whole-fat, fermented, raw (meaning not pasteurized or homogenized) dairy. Other people contend that dairy is one of the main culprits in the demise of Westerners' health.

**NUTRITION FACT**

Even though eggs are sometimes found in the dairy section of grocery stores, don't be confused: contrary to a pretty common misconception, eggs are not dairy products. Dairy is anything that is a product of the milk of a mammal, such as a cow, sheep, or goat.

Everyone agrees that before the advent of agriculture, people didn't consume milk after being weaned from their mothers, since milking a wild mastodon would have been a *little* tricky. Because we evolved to stop consuming it at a young age, it's not surprising that about 80 percent of the world becomes at least partially *lactose intolerant* during childhood.

**DEFINITION**

If you are **lactose intolerant,** that means you don't make the enzyme lactase to digest the lactose in milk. Raw milk contains lactase to help you digest it, but pasteurized milk doesn't.

There is evidence that dairy is one of the causes of many of our current health maladies, including digestive disorders, some cancers, insulin resistance, and acne. A small study published in 2005 in the *European Journal of Clinical Nutrition* showed that 8-year-old boys on a high-dairy diet developed significant insulin resistance. Insulin resistance is when your body doesn't respond to insulin, which is the hormone that allows glucose to be used and stored by your cells. Insulin resistance is the precursor to full-blown diabetes, and is thought to play a role in acne as well.

However, because those studies were almost all done using pasteurized, homogenized, low-fat, factory-farmed dairy products, part of the story is missing. There is evidence to support the health benefits of pasture-raised, whole-fat, raw milk products, including anticancer and antiacne effects. When milk is pasteurized, it's heated to kill harmful bacteria. However, that process also destroys good bacteria and rids the milk of many beneficial enzymes that help you use its nutrients. There is also another enzyme, lactase, in raw milk to help with the digestion of lactose. Raw milk is unpasteurized and unhomogenized, and it's something you can't find in grocery stores these days in the United States (except in California).

The jury is still out on dairy, partly because people all seem to react so differently to it. Our stance is that most people have a hard time digesting dairy to some extent, whether it be because of the lactose or the proteins in it. And even if you *can* digest it, the homogenization and pasteurization processes destroy much of the merit that raw dairy once had. Moreover, the extra estrogens in conventional milk affect hormone balance, contributing to who knows how many reproductive and other issues. It's advisable for you to go without dairy for at least a month to find out what kinds of effects, if any, dairy is having on you. After that time, if you choose to eat dairy, we strongly encourage you to consume only raw, whole-fat dairy from grass-fed animals, especially fermented products. We'll talk more about dairy in Chapter 3.

## Vegetable Oils

Fat is an incredibly important part of the human diet. Cell membranes, hormones, and brain function all depend on it. One thing is certain, though: hunter-gatherers didn't get their fat from corn, soy, or safflower oil. They ate the fat that comes from animals, tropical plants, fish, nuts, and seeds, and they rarely were overweight or died of heart disease.

The definition of "healthy fat" is a highly contentious, polarized topic in the nutrition world. The media and misinformed health professionals have the masses believing that saturated fat from animals and tropical oils causes heart disease. The American Heart Association and the American Dietetic Association want you to eat vegetable oil instead. But vegetable oils like soybean, safflower, sunflower, corn, and peanut oil are actually inferior foods that contribute to heart disease and inflammation of all kinds.

Western cultures have turned to vegetable oils, which are mostly comprised of poly-unsaturated fatty acids, because saturated fat has been demonized. However, some seriously flawed studies have been used to attack saturated fat. For instance, some negative studies on saturated fat actually used trans fats as their subject. Ironically, it's widely accepted now that trans fats, which are man-made saturated fats, contribute greatly to heart disease. Plus, new information has come out that disproves the idea that eating saturated fat and cholesterol causes heart disease. We lay rest to some of the myths about saturated fat and cholesterol in Chapter 4.

You may be wondering what all those fatty acids actually are—polyunsaturated, saturated, and trans fats. We explain more about these and other fatty acids in Chapters 4 and 8, but for now, here's how they break down:

- **Fatty acids**—The building blocks of fats and oils. They are constructed of a carboxylic acid with a long "tail" made mostly of carbon atoms. These long tails are either saturated by hydrogen, meaning they don't contain any double bonds, or they are unsaturated, meaning they contain one or more double bonds. All fatty acids are named according to the number of double bonds they contain.

- **Saturated fatty acids**—Fatty acids whose carbon chain is completely saturated by hydrogen and cannot absorb anymore hydrogen atoms. Saturated fat is generally solid at room temperature, and it's found in abundance in animal fats and tropical oils like coconut and palm. It's considered to be unhealthy by conventional standards, but recent research proves those claims to be false. (More on that in Chapter 4.)

- **Monounsaturated fatty acids**—These fatty acids have one double bond in their structure, hence *mono*. They are more susceptible to damage by heat, light, and oxygen than saturated fatty acids. They are found in foods like olive oil, lard, and other animal fat. They're considered to be heart-healthy fats, even by conventional standards. We agree.

- **Omega-3 fatty acids**—These are polyunsaturated fatty acids found in cold-water fish such as salmon and mackerel; certain nuts and seeds; and, in lesser amounts, leafy green vegetables. One of the double bonds is located on the third carbon atom from the end of the carbon chain, which is why it's called omega-*3*. These fatty acids are necessary to humans and they are anti-inflammatory.

- **Omega-6 fatty acids**—These are polyunsaturated fatty acids found abundantly in nuts and seeds. One of the double bonds is located on the sixth carbon atom from the end of the carbon chain, which is why it's called omega-*6*. These fatty acids are also necessary to humans, but they are inflammatory.

- **Polyunsaturated fatty acids**—These fatty acids have more than one double bond in their structure, hence the *poly*. They are liquid at room temperature and much more susceptible to damage by heat, air, and light than saturated or monounsaturated fats. Both omega-3s and omega-6s are polyunsaturated. They're found in abundance in cold-water fish, nuts and seeds, grains, and the oils of nuts and seeds. They're all considered to be healthy by conventional standards, but we now know that cooking with them can make them unhealthy, and that too many omega-6 fatty acids cause inflammation.

- **Trans fats**—These man-made fats are created by hydrogenating, or adding hydrogen molecules, to unsaturated fats. The process unnaturally turns unsaturated fats or oils into saturated ones in order to make them solid at room temperature and have a longer shelf life. It changes the structure into something unrecognizable by the body. Read the ingredients on bagged, canned, or other packaged foods and look for the word *hydrogenated*. If you see it, put the package down and walk away—those foods have been linked to heart disease and cancer.

So, contrary to conventional wisdom, it's not necessarily the saturated fat that's making us sick. Vegetable oils like corn, soy, safflower, sunflower, and cottonseed are contributing to our declining health, partly because of their high omega-6 fatty acid content. You may have heard of omega-6s before, probably in conjunction with omega-3 fatty acids. Omega-3s and omega-6s are both necessary for our bodies, but we don't make them ourselves so we have to get them from food. A big difference between them is that omega-3s *decrease* inflammation, while too many omega-6s *increase* chronic inflammation. Chronic inflammation contributes to everything from achy joints to obesity, asthma, irritable bowel disease, diabetes, and heart disease.

**NUTRITION FACT**

You may be shocked to learn that most vegetable oil is not only highly processed with high heat and a petroleum-derived solvent, but it also must be deodorized as a final step because of the rancid smell.

In order to keep the inflammation at bay, you need a healthy ratio of omega-6 to omega-3—somewhere between 1:1 and 4:1. The current ratio in the typical Western diet has skyrocketed to around 20:1—and sometimes up to 45:1—because of vegetable oils and grains. Compared to our ancestors, people are eating way too many omega-6s and not enough omega-3s. It's ironic that they're called vegetable oils because they're not made of vegetables. Some of them aren't even made of edible plant matter, like cottonseed oil.

Where are people getting these vegetable oils? According to the U.S. Bureau of Labor Statistics, people are spending a monumental 40 percent of their food dollars at restaurants, up from only 3 percent in 1901. Most of the oils in restaurants are vegetable oils, which are highly refined and/or hydrogenated. Not only that, but vegetable oils are usually chemically treated and stripped of almost all their nutrients. They're empty calories, just like the refined grains and sugars.

Even if you're not going out to eat, the packaged foods you buy in grocery stores very often use corn oil, soybean oil, sunflower oil, canola oil, and safflower oil. We'll talk more about canola oil—which, despite its reputation as a healthy oil, isn't much better than other vegetable oils—in Chapter 3.

**PALEO COMPASS**

Some unrefined, high-quality plant oils are acceptable on the Paleolithic diet, such as extra-virgin olive oil, virgin coconut oil, virgin palm oil, avocado oil, and some nut oils. Olive oil is mostly a monounsaturated fat, and therefore doesn't contribute much to the inflammation-promoting omega-6 to omega-3 ratio. Coconut oil is mostly saturated, so it's totally acceptable. And some nut oils, like macadamia, have a favorable fatty acid composition.

## Unnecessary Additives

Another major difference in our modern diet is that Paleolithic people didn't add yellow #5 or artificial sweeteners to their food. There were no synthetic preservatives like sulfites, potassium sorbate, or disodium EDTA. There were no fluorescent-colored sports drinks, artificially flavored gummy worms, or brominated wheat flour. Luckily for them, they didn't have the technology to make artificial flavorings, colorings, preservatives, bulking agents, or sweeteners (or any of the other 19 categories of food additives we have now).

While some food additives are harmless, many have been tested and shown to be toxic in some way. For instance, the preservative sodium benzoate is found in carbonated drinks, salad dressings, and even pharmaceuticals, and when combined with other common food additives it has been linked with cancer and ADHD. Others, such as nitrates and aspartame, have been linked with digestive problems, migraines, neurological conditions, heart disease, and obesity.

Children are often especially susceptible to the effects of synthetic additives because their brains and other tissues are still developing. That makes it even more alarming that the most brightly colored, preservative-rich products like Gatorade, colored cereals, and candy are being marketed directly to children.

Unfortunately, when you read the ingredient lists of most of the prepackaged, processed foods that come from conventional grocery stores, you will find a host of additives. They're also found in conventional deli meats, nuts, dried fruit, and other foods you might call all-natural if you didn't first read the ingredients.

It's common to think that in such small quantities these ingredients aren't going to hurt you, yet over a lifetime of eating them every day many will take their toll.

## The Least You Need to Know

- You can lose weight and enjoy better health overall by eating the foods our Paleolithic ancestors ate.
- The foods Paleolithic people ate that gave them such vibrant health were wild animals, fruits, vegetables, and some nuts and seeds.
- People's health declined with the advent of agriculture and the consumption of grains, legumes, pasteurized dairy, refined sugar, vegetable oils, and additives.
- Returning to a diet that mimics our ancestors is a simple and logical way to increase your health and reverse a general trend toward obesity and sickness.

# Benefits of Eating Paleo

## In This Chapter

- Better for your digestion
- Slim down and kick diabetes
- Stay energized and happy every day
- Improve your athletic performance
- Teeming with nutrients
- Clear, glowing skin

There are benefits to many diets, but the Paleo way of eating combines all those virtues into one superior, sustainable diet. For instance, the raw foods diet is great for its nutrient-rich, whole plant foods, but it lacks enough protein for many people. The Atkins diet recognizes that too many carbohydrates cause weight gain, but it allows for pasteurized dairy and highly processed foods. Even the new guidelines from the USDA tout fruits and vegetables as being more important than ever, but they still push for a lot of grains (even refined grains), low-fat pasteurized dairy, and vegetable oils. This chapter highlights how the Paleolithic diet can change your health and life more thoroughly and sustainably than any other diet out there.

## Better Digestion

When people change their diet to incorporate Paleo versus non-Paleo foods, they're often surprised by how quickly their digestive problems, like bloating, heartburn, and gas, go away. You often don't realize how bad your digestive symptoms are until they're gone. People also think that feeling bloated after every meal or having gas is just the way life is, but those things are not normal, much less healthy, parts of life.

But gut health goes beyond just the obvious gas, bloating, constipation, diarrhea, or stomach cramps: your gut has a lot to do with inflammation and nutrient absorption, too, which affect your overall health. As we mentioned in Chapter 1, there are harmful substances found in non-Paleo foods, like lectins, phytates, and gluten. Let's take a closer look at how all of them affect your gut, and your health, in various ways.

## Lectins

Lectins are proteins found in animals (including you) and plants. They're everywhere, especially in grains, legumes (especially soy), nuts, and seeds.

> **DAMAGE CONTROL**
>
> Because nuts and seeds contain some of the antinutrients lectins and phytic acid, their presence in the Paleolithic diet has been questioned. We suggest that you limit your nuts and seeds to 1 or 2 ounces per day. Better yet, sprout or soak your nuts and seeds to remove most of the antinutrients. See Chapter 3 for more information.

Lectins live in the seeds of plants, like grains and legumes, and can cause considerable intestinal distress (diarrhea, nausea, bloating, vomiting, and even death) to those who eat too many of the seeds, perhaps in hopes of deterring the predator (you) from coming back for more. So it takes a considerable amount of preparing and cooking to make grains and legumes digestible and palatable at all. Although cooking, sprouting, or soaking grains and legumes helps decrease the amount of lectins they contain, none of those processes completely eliminates them.

### Immune Response

Wheat contains a particular lectin called wheat germ agglutinin, or WGA. Lectins are sticky little buggers, and the WGA goes into your small intestine and gloms onto its lining. It then tricks your body into taking it across the border of your intestine intact, where it's seen as a foreign invader by your immune system.

Antibodies are created in response to the lectins, and unfortunately, lectins often look a lot like other parts of your body. They may look like cells in your brain, pancreas, etc., so the same antibodies that were created to attack the lectin will actually go launch attacks on *your own body*. Some studies show that this process could contribute to autoimmune issues, like rheumatoid arthritis, celiac disease, lupus, and multiple sclerosis.

**Leaky Gut and Food Sensitivities**

To make things worse, on their way into your body, lectins damage the walls of your intestines, helping to create "leaky gut." Leaky gut happens when the tight junctions of the intestines are damaged, allowing large particles to cross the intestinal barrier, enter your bloodstream, and stimulate immune responses.

In other words, something (like the WGA) damages your gut, which allows big particles of food into your bloodstream. Your immune system then gets overwhelmed and confused and starts attacking foods at random, even foods that would otherwise be healthy for us. This is how *food sensitivities* manifest. Leaky gut and food sensitivities symptoms may include, among other things, digestive problems, headaches, eczema, anxiety, fatigue, seasonal allergies, acne, and possibly even autism and type 1 diabetes.

**DEFINITION**

**Food sensitivities** are negative immune responses to a certain food.

Food sensitivities can be diagnosed by a blood or stool test. It's different than testing for food allergies with your allergist, though. True food "allergies" are mitigated by immunoglobulin E, a particular part of your immune system. Most conventional doctors don't know that it's possible to test for other immune responses besides immunoglobulin E. However, other parts of the immune system, like prostaglandins, histamine, and cytokines, can be involved in a response to foods—not just immunoglobulin E. When it's not immunoglobulin E doing the work, then it's called a food "sensitivity" as opposed to an allergy. Talk to a naturopath or a nutritionist about getting tested for food sensitivities. When you figure out which foods are triggering your immune system, you can stop eating them for a while to help improve your symptoms and heal.

# Phytic Acid (Phytates)

Phytic acid, also called phytate or phytates, is another antinutrient found in grains and legumes. Unfortunately, phytates aren't digestible by nonruminants (read: non-cud-chewers) because we lack the enzyme phytase to break them down. What's bad about phytates is that they bind to magnesium, calcium, zinc, and iron in your intestines and excrete those vital nutrients from your body. What does that mean for your overall health?

- Some experts believe that phytates' ability to bind with iron is greatly contributing to the worldwide epidemic of iron-deficiency anemia.

- Magnesium deficiency can contribute to everything from muscle cramping to PMS to insomnia and anxiety.

- Zinc is incredibly important to the immune system and for reproductive abilities, so any deficiency could wreak havoc on our health.

- Calcium deficiency can cause fragile bones, tooth decay, insomnia, and anxiety.

The good news is that you can sprout, ferment, and soak most of the phytates out of just about anything, but those practices have been all but laid to rest in the modern world.

## Gluten

Gluten is another harmful substance that is in some grains. It's a protein that acts like glue (hence its name) in baked goods, giving them the doughy consistency everybody loves. Nowadays, it's also found as an additive in everything from ice cream to ketchup.

Going gluten free is becoming more and more common because so many people feel better without it. Gluten is found in the following grains and the foods made from them:

- Barley

- Kamut (another ancient wheat relative)

- Oats (from cross contamination with wheat)

- Rye

- Spelt (an ancient relative of wheat)

- Wheat (durum, triticale, couscous, semolina, etc.)

It's believed that anywhere from 30 to 75 percent of the population have a sensitivity to gluten. The symptoms include headaches, fatigue, skin rash, asthma, joint pain, acid reflux, abdominal cramping, diarrhea, and intense cravings.

You may have heard of celiac disease, which is an autoimmune disorder caused by gluten. The immune system attacks cells of the small intestine when it mistakes them for gliadin, a protein in gluten. Symptoms are fatigue, digestive disturbances, and nutrient deficiencies. About 1 percent of the Western world has been diagnosed with celiac disease, but many more people are thought to have it.

With so many digestive problems with grains and legumes, it seems almost obvious that we didn't evolve eating them. Taking them off the menu is one of the paramount benefits of the Paleolithic diet.

## Lactose Intolerance

As we mentioned in Chapter 1, another major digestive culprit is lactose, the sugar found in milk. Do you ever get bloating or terrible gas after eating ice cream or drinking milk? Maybe even diarrhea? That could be lactose intolerance. Genetic research shows that most hunter-gatherer societies, Paleolithic and modern, were lactose intolerant after being weaned from their mothers. Over the last 10,000 years, certain groups who depended highly on milk developed genetic mutations that allowed them to continue to produce lactase; they evolved. Many people now still carry those mutated genes, but often only to a certain degree.

> **PALEO COMPASS**
>
> The Dutch and Danes, who have a long history of consuming dairy products, have the lowest rates of lactose intolerance. Alaskan Eskimos and Thais, who haven't consumed much dairy at all in their history, are some of the most lactose intolerant people of the world.

Some people, depending on their genetic makeup and gut health, might do just fine with certain dairy products. Overall, though, many people have issues with it, for obvious evolutionary reasons: people didn't drink milk after they were weaned until 10,000 years ago. It's recommended that you remove dairy from your diet for a month when you start the diet to see if your digestive health improves. You may be surprised to find that you're one of the many lactose-intolerant people of the world. (See Chapter 3 for more about dairy products.)

# Lose Fat, Gain Muscle, Fight Diabetes

If weight loss is your main goal with the switch to Paleo, then you're in luck: people who go from eating a typical Western diet to a Paleolithic diet usually lose fat and gain muscle. However, if your goal is to bulk up and gain muscle mass, eating Paleo is a great way to do that, too. As a bonus of changing your diet and body composition, the signs and symptoms of diabetes also diminish.

## Weight Loss

Weight loss can be a lifelong struggle for people. The battle of the bulge is often a lot of sacrifice (and hunger) with little payoff. There are low-fat diets, very low-carb diets, no-meat diets, and extremely low-calorie diets that are all designed to help you lose weight.

People can only resist cravings for fat, *carbohydrates*, meat, or calories for so long, until at some point they find their hand involuntarily opening a bag of cookies or a pint of ice cream.

**DEFINITION**

**Carbohydrates** are one of the three macronutrients that provide calories, the others being protein and fat. They can be simple sugars like glucose and fructose or more complex sugars like starch and fiber. Carbohydrates are found in abundance in grains (such as flour, bread, and pasta), refined sugars, legumes, vegetables, and fruits. Your body uses carbohydrates as energy for your muscles and organs, although it can also use fat and protein.

When you're trying to lose weight, deprivation doesn't work in the long run, but eating moderate amounts of the foods you were designed to eat will keep extra weight off forever. That's why so many people consider eating Paleo a way of life and not just a diet. Good fats, lots of protein, and Paleo carbs (fruits and vegetables) are incredibly satisfying, unlike prepackaged meals you might get on some diet plans that leave you craving something more.

### Water Retention

Sometimes people lose enormous amounts of weight when they first start eating Paleo because they're dropping water weight. Eating a lot of carbohydrates makes you retain water because your body assumes that you'll need that water when you're doing physical work later, burning off the carbs. But if you don't exercise to get rid of the excess sugar (and the extra water), you can end up carrying around a lot of unneces-sary water weight. That water often takes the form of puffy eyes, edema in your legs, or swollen feet. If you find yourself making extra trips to the bathroom when you first start eating Paleo, don't worry! It's just the extra water (and weight) making its way out.

Water retention can also be caused by food sensitivities or allergies. People are com-monly sensitive or allergic to grains, legumes (particularly soy), sugar, and dairy. Eating Paleo gets rid of all of those foods, giving your immune system a much-needed break, and allowing the water to flush out.

### Carbohydrates and Weight Loss

After the water weight is gone, you might still have some extra body fat to contend with. A lot of the success of this diet comes from removing empty-calorie carbohy-drate foods like refined sugar and refined grains from your life. Extra carbs create excess glucose in your bloodstream. If that glucose isn't used up quickly, it gets stored as glycogen for later. And if that's not used up during exercise later, it's stored as fat.

## Diabetes

Having glucose in the bloodstream is actually toxic to your body, so insulin is there to open the gates to your cells so that they can use the glucose or store it. Insulin is basically a key to your cells. When there's too much sugar in your blood for too long, though, your body can become insulin resistant. That's when the cells lose receptor sites for insulin, so the insulin can't do its job of letting glucose into the cells. Glucose ends up toxically remaining in the bloodstream, eventually causing diabetes.

In order to manage—not cure—diabetes, diabetics are told by mainstream medicine to take insulin or other pharmaceuticals, and to eat whole grains and low-fat every-thing because of the fear of animal fats and high protein. What actually needs to happen is the removal of all foods that cause a high glucose spike in the bloodstream: grains, beans, and sugar. *That* is how people reverse diabetes and get off their medications.

The goal is not necessarily to take out all carbohydrates, though. That's not sustain-able or necessary for most people. However, blood sugar is one of the most important aspects of weight loss and diabetes, and if you don't get it under control, you're going to have a hard time taking off the pounds and regaining your health. Eating Paleo is a balance of eating enough good carbohydrates in the form of vegetables and fruits and removing the blood glucose–spiking carbohydrate sources like sugar, bread, pasta, and other grain products. Those foods are unnecessary and only cause unnecessary blood glucose spikes, which perpetuate diabetes.

## Putting on Muscle Mass

The pictures of body builders' bulging muscles on the labels of protein powders should have tipped you off about the fact that *protein* builds muscle. That's why when people eat Paleo, they often start to see more muscle tone. This diet is up to 35 percent protein, which is a lot compared to the 15 percent in the average Western diet.

**DEFINITION**

**Protein** is a macronutrient (one of three: protein, carbohydrates, and fat) composed of amino acids, which are made of nitrogen, carbon, and oxygen. High-protein foods include meat and organs, fish, eggs, dairy, and nuts, in that order. You need protein for muscle and bone growth, and to repair and heal damaged tissue, among many other functions.

You can see results on the diet even without lifting enormous weights every day, and it's because muscle growth is fueled by protein. Basically, if you feed them protein, they'll grow. Even if you didn't do any exercise at all (which is not advisable), you would likely see more muscle tone on this diet. Many people have done just that.

That doesn't necessarily mean that you'll bulk up, though. Most women don't want giant quadriceps that don't fit in their jeans, and that's probably not what's going to happen. We're just saying that there's a good chance you'll replace some of that extra fat with lean muscle. Here's how.

Protein, along with fat, satiates hunger and curbs cravings for sugar between meals. Think about it: have you ever eaten a high-carb meal like pasta with veggies (with no meat) and felt cravings for cookies an hour later—heck, 15 minutes later? If you eat the same number of calories in the form of meat, studies have shown that people eat less later.

Protein also requires a lot of energy to digest and assimilate, meaning your body has to burn calories in order to gain energy from dietary protein. In other words, it boosts your metabolism—way more than fat or carbohydrates do.

So while protein builds and repairs your muscles to give you the svelte body you've always wanted, it also keeps your sugar and calorie intake in check, helping you lose fat. It's a win-win situation. Plus, muscle doesn't just look better than fat: Muscle cell insulin receptors are also much more efficient than fat cell insulin receptors, and that's a good thing.

# Blood Sugar, Mood, and Energy

We're emphasizing blood sugar because it really is one of the biggest problems with the modern diet. Because we evolved to take advantage of simple sugars when we could get our hands on them, a lot of us lack self-control around foods like pastries and cookies. It's not entirely your fault when you eat the whole pan of brownies before you have the chance to bring them to your office. We are products of our environment, and we live in an environment that caters to our instinctive sugar cravings.

But giving in to those cravings every day can affect your mood and energy levels. It's easier to resist the temptation of sugar, and thereby have more balanced moods and more energy every day, when you know exactly what it's doing to your body.

## Understanding Blood Sugar

Because sugar is the simplest food to break down, our bodies naturally crave it when we're in a low blood sugar state of desperation—feeling hungry, irritable, shaky, and light-headed. The good and bad news is that sugar begets sugar cravings. That's because if you spike your blood sugar with refined grains, sugar, or caffeine, that upward feeling of jittery energy will quickly be followed by a downward plunge when your blood sugar drops. All that sugar was scooped up out of your bloodstream into your cells for storage, and you have a blood sugar crash: you might feel fatigued, grumpy, depressed, light-headed, or have a headache.

This feeling can happen whether or not you've had sugar recently—it's basically your body telling you you're hungry. But the blood sugar crashes happen way more often, and are more intense, when you're constantly eating sugary foods. That's because those foods create a quick drop in blood sugar—a high spike followed by an equally low plunge. When you're eating sufficient protein, fat, and fiber to mitigate those plunges, it just doesn't happen as often. Your body can turn protein and fat into glucose if it needs to. By eating those foods, along with Paleo sources of carbs, your blood sugar stays more even, until the steady stream of energy is depleted and you actually need to eat.

## Cortisol to the Rescue

When your blood sugar gets too low, *cortisol* comes to save the day by asking your liver and muscles to put some much-needed glucose into your blood to keep you on your feet. Unfortunately, too much cortisol also disarms the immune system, stops bone growth, and hinders the reproductive system.

> **DEFINITION**
>
> **Cortisol** is a hormone produced and secreted by the adrenal glands in response to low blood sugar or other stressful situations. Its main purpose is to tell the liver and muscles to secrete glucose into the bloodstream.

The good news is that there's a system in place to keep you alive if you run out of food. The bad news is that if cortisol is being overused every day, it can lead to belly fat, immune suppression, reproductive issues, mood disorders, and chronic fatigue, among many other things. When you get to that low blood sugar place, epinephrine (or adrenaline) is also released, because your body sees a lack of food as a stressful situation. Chronically high levels of epinephrine can contribute to anxiety, chronic fatigue, and high blood pressure, among other things.

So blood sugar swings obviously cause short-term mood and energy swings, but they also have more serious effects on your health in the long term. The way to stop the vicious cycle of blood sugar spikes and crashes is to eat a Paleolithic diet. It keeps your blood sugar steady, and cortisol and epinephrine in check.

# Enhanced Athletic Performance

For all the reasons we've just discussed, the Paleolithic diet will help with your athletic endeavors. Nobody can perform their best when they're chronically fatigued or battling anxiety. And blood sugar roller-coaster rides won't get you through a long workout, much less an intense race or other competitive event. Beyond that, though, a Paleolithic diet can improve athletic performance by getting you to your optimal body composition and decreasing joint pain.

## Optimal Body Composition

When you're at your ideal weight, you're going to run faster or jump higher than if you're 40 pounds overweight. And because there's more protein in this diet to create muscle, you'll naturally be stronger. The protein also helps repair your muscles and tissues, so your recovery time will be shorter, too.

## Joint Pain

Joint pain can be devastating to an athlete. Pain comes from inflammation, and that inflammation often stems from food. Your immune system reacts to food particles that cross through the gut lining due to leaky gut (discussed earlier in this chapter). Cytokines and other parts of your immune system can create inflammation and increase the amount of pain you feel. The omega-6 to omega-3 balance is also paramount in keeping inflammation under control, which is easy when you're eating Paleo.

We all experience normal amounts of inflammation, especially if we're athletic. It's a natural part of muscles breaking down and then recovering. But when inflammation becomes chronic from things like food sensitivities and overconsumption of omega-6 fatty acids, it can lead to many health problems, like joint pain.

# A Nutrient-Dense Diet

Without whole grains, beans, and dairy, you might be wondering how you'll get all the vitamins and minerals you need. Think of it like this: instead of the empty, filler foods like refined flour and sugar that hog space in the typical Western diet, you'll only be eating foods that are brimming with nutrients. And because the bulk of your diet will no longer contain phytic acid, which inhibits absorption of crucial minerals, you get to *keep* the nutrients you eat.

If you think of every time you eat as an opportunity to extract vital nutrients from food, then it seems wasteful to eat things like white bread or corn syrup. Refined foods like that, even though they're sometimes re-injected with synthetic vitamins and minerals, can deplete your own nutrient stores. If the foods on your daily menu are mostly high-quality animal foods, fresh vegetables and fruits, and some nuts, you're always adding to your nutrient cache.

Two recent studies showed that lean meats, fish, vegetables, and fruit are significantly better sources than whole grains and dairy of the 13 vitamins and minerals most lacking in the Western diet.

Let's talk a bit about one nutrient in particular that a lot of Paleo naysayers have an issue with. You may be wondering whether or not you'll get enough calcium on this diet without dairy. The short answer is yes. Let's take a closer look at the long answer.

## The Calcium Paradox

There's a calcium craze going on right now. Western adults and children alike are eating dairy like it's their job, hoping to get enough calcium to avoid the scourge of brittle bones. On top of that, people are supplementing with calcium chews and pills to fulfill the lofty RDA of around 1,000 milligrams of calcium per day. Despite all this, osteoporosis rates are not decreasing. In fact, according to the Centers for Disease Control and Prevention (CDC), 49 percent of women and 30 percent of men over 50 in the United States suffer from osteopenia, which is defined as reduced bone mass of lesser severity than osteoporosis. That's 22.7 million women in the United States alone who are well on their way to osteoporosis. Approximately 10 percent of women in the United States over 50 have osteoporosis. This is a large, looming problem. About 20 percent of people who sustain osteoporotic spine or hip fractures die within 12 months. And most people require full assistance, meaning they lose most independence, to recover from spine or hip fractures.

So what's wrong with just taking calcium and eating dairy to build bones? It actually takes many nutrients—not just calcium—plus protein, weight-bearing exercise, estrogen, and sunlight (vitamin D) to grow your bones. Plus, even though dairy contains a lot of calcium, so do edible fish bones (such as are in canned salmon and sardines), dark leafy green vegetables, and nuts.

The most important thing about calcium consumption is that you keep what you eat. Dairy is an acid-forming food in your body, just like grains and legumes, but calcium requires an alkaline environment to be absorbed properly. So if your body is acidic you will leach calcium from your bones and excrete it in your urine. Goodbye calcium. That is the paradox: eating dairy could actually reduce the calcium in your body. Here's another paradox: some calcium supplements are full of sugar, artificial flavors and colors, corn syrup, and milk. Just one more reason to always read the labels on everything!

Another way you lose calcium is by eating phytates in grains, legumes, and nuts, which bind to calcium in your intestines and carry it out unabsorbed. To make things worse, taking in too much calcium can inhibit the absorption of magnesium, another very important nutrient for bone and muscle health.

## Tips for Building Strong Bones

The following are some things you and your children can do for optimal bone health, besides eating a Paleolithic diet. All of these are common traits of a hunter-gatherer lifestyle:

- Get out in the sun every day and/or take a vitamin $D_3$ supplement. Vitamin $D_3$ is necessary for calcium absorption.

- Avoid chronic stress and blood sugar imbalances. Your body creates cortisol in response to both of those things, and cortisol inhibits bone growth.

- Do weight bearing exercise (such as weight lifting, rock climbing, any resistance training exercises, hiking, or stair climbing) at least three times a week. Muscle pulling on bone builds bone.

- Go easy on caffeine—it increases calcium excretion.

- If you insist on taking a supplement for bone health, purchase a multimineral and multivitamin supplement from a nutrition practitioner that includes all the necessary nutrients for building bones.

# Improved Skin Health

You can use abrasive antimicrobial cleansers, take antibiotics, ingest hormone pills, or apply corticosteroids to your skin to ward off unwanted acne and rashes. Or you can eat Paleo. Skin problems usually don't stem from something outside your body like dirt or bacteria; they are actually a sign of problems on the inside.

The same way leaky gut can cause joint pain, it can cause skin problems, too. The immune response that leaky gut causes can manifest in many ways, including acne, eczema, psoriasis, dermatitis, and many others. We've all heard that chocolate causes acne. Well, that may be true if chocolate is one of the things your particular body is sensitive to, but it could also be grains, dairy, or any other foods causing the immune response. It depends on the person.

Removing the non-Paleo foods helps your gut heal. When you're not eating harmful foods every day (or every meal) that are causing leaky gut, your intestinal lining can mend itself and your immune system can calm down. In the process, your skin will clear up and you'll be able to throw away all those expensive, abrasive pharmaceuticals and cleansers.

## The Least You Need to Know

- Some antinutrients, like lectins, phytates, and gluten in non-Paleo foods can cause major digestive disorders and immune reactions.
- The high protein and relatively low carbohydrate content of the Paleolithic diet keep you satisfied while helping you lose weight and gain muscle.
- Without the blood sugar spikes and common food sensitivities of a normal Western diet, the Paleolithic diet keeps your mood and energy levels even.
- Athletic performance benefits from more muscle, optimal body weight, high energy levels, and less joint and muscle pain—all attainable through the Paleolithic diet.
- The Paleolithic diet contains all the nutrients you need, including calcium.
- Beautiful, clear skin starts with great digestive health, and the Paleolithic diet does a belly good.

# What to Eat (and Not to Eat)

## In This Chapter

- Foods you should eat often
- Foods you should sometimes eat
- Foods you should run from
- Foods up for debate

In this chapter, we give you some guidelines for what foods are and are not part of a Paleolithic diet. This guide is a culmination of what we know about what our ancestors ate, what modern hunter-gatherers thrive on, and current research and opinions. With opinions come disagreements, though, so there are a handful of foods that are hotly debated in the Paleo community. We'll give you the information you need to make your own decisions about foods like canola oil, dairy, potatoes, and diet sodas. Many of the debates are just products of outdated research, so we'll update you.

# Acceptable Paleo Foods

For all the categories that follow, it's optimal to eat organic- and pasture-raised foods if you can afford to or have access to them. The nutrient value is generally higher in those foods, and pesticides and other nonorganic practices can be harmful to our health and to the environment.

## Vegetables

You can eat as many vegetables as your heart desires, except for starchy vegetables: cassava (tapioca and manioc), potatoes, sweet potatoes, taro, yucca, and yams. Eat starchy veggies no more than 1 to 3 days per week if you're trying to lose weight and lower your blood glucose levels. Eat them in moderation (2 to 5 days per week) if you exercise regularly and are trying to lose weight. If you are a very active endurance athlete, you may need to eat them on a more regular basis. We discuss the Paleo athlete's diet in more detail in Chapter 6.

**DAMAGE CONTROL**

The nightshade family (potatoes, bell peppers, chili peppers, paprika, eggplants, tomatoes, and tobacco) may provoke symptoms in people with autoimmune disorders or leaky gut. Eat at your own discretion.

## Fruits

Eat fruits freely, unless you're trying to lose weight. In that case, limit daily fruit intake to one or two servings, especially dried fruit (no more than 2 ounces).

Eating a lot of fructose, the main sugar in fruits, can lead to weight gain, heart disease, high blood pressure, and kidney disease. On average, Paleolithic man most likely ate between 15 to 25 grams of fructose per day, and only when it was seasonally available. Our bodies did not evolve processing much fructose. Today the average American consumes 70 to 80 grams of fructose a day, mainly in the form of high-fructose corn syrup. For optimal health and quick weight loss, you should limit your intake to 25 to 30 grams a day from any source.

## Meats and Eggs

In order to mimic our ancestors best, eat products from animals that were grass fed, pasture raised, or found in the wild. Meat from those animals contains a less inflammatory fatty acid profile, which we talk about more in Chapter 4.

Don't forget about the organs! While not typically part of a fast-food culture, organ meats and bone marrow were prized by hunter-gatherers for their high nutrient content. For instance, brains contain high amounts of omega-3 fatty acids, bone marrow is full of heart-healthy monounsaturated fatty acids, and liver provides an abundance of vitamin A. Whale skin even provided Inuits with vital vitamin C to get them through the winters. Organs are high in protein, too.

Steer clear of meats with preservatives and color or flavor enhancers, particularly added nitrites, as they have been linked with stomach cancer. Often it's the processed meats like bacon, sausage, hot dogs, beef jerky, and deli meats that contain those added ingredients. If you buy those meats from a health food store or a local source, you'll be able to avoid the unwanted ingredients. As for eggs, if you can't find pasture-raised eggs, buy omega-3 eggs.

All cuts of meat are acceptable on this diet, but try to vary them as much as possible. Each part of the animal contains different levels of protein and beneficial fatty acids that you should take advantage of. In other words, as delicious as bacon may be, don't make it your only animal protein!

Meats to include:

- Beef
- Buffalo
- Chicken
- Game meats
- Goat
- Lamb
- Organs and marrow
- Pork
- Turkey

**NUTRITION FACT**

Eggs (especially from pasture-raised chickens) are a good source of choline, which is a brain nutrient, lutein for your eyes, and many other vitamins and minerals. They're also a source of vitamin D, which many people are deficient in. The yolks are where you'll find the bulk of the nutrients, so don't throw them away! And their protein is found in the white *and* in the yolk: another reason to eat the whole egg.

## Fish, Shellfish, and Fish Eggs

All species are acceptable, but we recommend you research the mercury and other pollutant levels of your favorite fish. According to the Natural Resources Defense Council (NRDC), the fish highest in mercury are bluefish, grouper, mackerel (Spanish, king, and gulf), marlin, orange roughy, sea bass, shark, swordfish, and tuna (bigeye, yellowfin, and canned albacore). The fish lowest in mercury include anchovies, catfish, clams, crabs, crawfish, herring, mackerel (North Atlantic and chub), salmon (canned and wild-caught), sardines, shrimp, tilapia, and trout.

The NRDC website (nrdc.org) is an excellent resource for researching mercury levels. The Monterey Bay Aquarium (montereybayaquarium.org) also has very good information on the environmental impact of different kinds of fish farms and fishing practices.

Wild-caught fish and seafood are generally better than farm-raised for high nutrient and lower pollutant content. Many fish have high levels of omega-3 fatty acids that contribute to a healthy omega-6 to omega-3 ratio.

Fish and seafood to include:

- All fish eggs
- Anchovies
- Bass
- Cod
- Crab
- Eel
- Flatfish
- Halibut
- Mahi mahi
- Monkfish
- Salmon
- Sardines
- Shrimp
- Walleye

## Nuts and Seeds

Note that peanuts are not nuts; they're legumes, so they're not on this list. Soaking and sprouting nuts and seeds can remove much of their antinutrient content. All of the following nuts and seeds, plus their flours and butters, are totally acceptable.

However, nuts and seeds are high in calories: a cup of almonds contains about 822 calories! For comparison, a cup of blueberries provides 84 calories, and a cup of avocado is 384 calories. This is a good reason to limit your intake of nuts and seeds to 1 or 2 ounces a day, especially in the beginning if you're trying to lose weight.

Nuts and seeds to include:

- Almonds
- Brazil nuts
- Cashews
- Chestnuts
- Flaxseeds and flax meal
- Hazelnuts
- Macadamias
- Pecans
- Pine nuts
- Pistachio
- Pumpkin seeds
- Sesame seeds
- Sunflower seeds
- Walnuts

## Sea Vegetables

All sea vegetables are an excellent source of vitamins and minerals and they add tons of flavor to foods. You can slice them up and put them in soups, eat them dried as snacks, or use nori as a substitute for a sandwich wrap.

Sea vegetables to include:

- Kombu
- Hijiki
- Nori
- Wakame

## Fats and Oils

All of the oils and fats on this list should be extra-virgin, virgin, and/or unrefined if possible. The more refined an oil is, the more heat it's been exposed to and the fewer nutrients it contains.

Fats and oils to include:

- Avocado oil
- Coconut oil
- Coconut milk (see the following sidebar)
- Flaxseed oil (see discussion later in this chapter)
- Hazelnut oil
- Lard
- Macadamia oil
- Olive oil
- Sesame oil
- Tallow
- Unrefined palm oil
- Walnut oil

> **PALEO COMPASS**
>
> Don't confuse *coconut milk,* which is found in a soup-sized can and made from coconut flesh and water, with *coconut water,* which is the water that comes out of a young coconut and sold as a canned beverage. The coconut milk on the previous list also does not mean the coconut "milk" that comes in a container like soy milk or almond milk, which is made from coconut flesh, a lot of water, and some added thickeners and nutrients. Both coconut water and coconut "milk" are acceptable on the diet, although they don't contain much fat.

## Beverages

For the most part, stick with filtered or spring water to drink: tap water often contains pollutants and chlorine, which can be harmful to your digestive system. After all, chlorine is meant to kill bacteria, and there's beneficial bacteria in your gut that you don't want to kill off. Most other drinks contain sweeteners and chemical additives and lack nutrients due to heavy processing.

Beverages to include:

- Coconut water

- Filtered or spring water

- Herbal tea

## Herbs and Spices

All herbs and spices are totally acceptable, including a minimal amount of unrefined sea salt (but not refined, iodized salt; see the later section). Make sure you read the ingredient lists in spice mixes: sometimes they have corn or other unnecessary additives in them.

# Consume in Moderation

You may be wondering what "in moderation" means. These are some of the foods and beverages that are debatable in the Paleo community, and each has its own guidelines. Read the "Is It Paleo or Not?" section later in this chapter for more information on the following:

- Alcohol

- Caffeinated teas

- Coffee

- Dark chocolate

- Sweeteners (raw honey, coconut sap, stevia)

- Vinegar

# Foods to Avoid

The foods discussed in the following sections are what you should try to avoid. Of course, there will be "cheats" here and there, but the majority of your meals should not contain them.

## Grains or Grainlike Foods

Avoid any of the following grains as well as any flours, pastas, noodles, breads, cookies, crackers, bagels, pastries, or other foods made from them. White flour is actually just refined wheat flour, so it is also a no-no. For a full list of what products contain grains, see Chapter 7.

Gluten grains to avoid:

- Barley

- Oats

- Rye

- Spelt

- Wheat

Nongluten grains to avoid:

- Amaranth

- Buckwheat

- Bulgar

- Corn

- Millet

- Quinoa

- Rice

- Sorghum

- Teff

**PALEO COMPASS**

You may be wondering how you'll ever enjoy anything breadlike again if you don't eat that ever-present white (made from wheat) flour. Paleo eaters still love baked goods, so we make delicious and nutritious muffins, cookies, and breads out of almond flour, coconut flour, and tapioca flour. See Chapter 8 for more on using these flours.

## Legumes (Beans)

Legumes are anything that comes from the pod of the *Leguminosae* family of plants. In other words, beans. Soy is a legume, and it's in a lot of products, so watch out for anything that says "soy" in the ingredient list. It's slipped into everything from cookies to marinara sauces in the form of soy protein, soy lecithin, soy oil, and others.

Avoid the following legumes, as well as any flour, crackers, tofu, milk, sauce, butter, or other product made from these foods:

- Adzuki beans
- Black beans
- Garbanzo beans
- Lentils
- Lima beans
- Mung beans
- Navy beans
- Peanuts
- Peas
- Pinto beans
- Red beans
- Soy (edamame, soy flour, tofu, tempeh, soy sauce, tamari, soy milk)

**PALEO COMPASS**

Common vegetables like snow peas and green beans are actually legumes because they're found in a pod. However, they are generally acceptable on the Paleolithic diet. The young seeds of those foods contain fewer antinutrients than the older, dried-out seeds of non-Paleo foods like lentils or soy. Plus, they aren't generally eaten in large quantities. Go ahead and enjoy those pod veggies.

## Refined and Artificial Sweeteners

Almost everyone loves sweet foods. In fact, when one hunter-gatherer group in Africa was asked which of their commonly eaten foods they preferred, most men and women chose honey. But humans generally evolved eating only limited seasonal raw honey and potentially coconut sap. Our bodies aren't well equipped to handle refined sugars in copious amounts. They cause blood sugar spikes, and we don't want that. There will probably be times when these slip into your diet, but try to stick with the lowest glycemic index sweeteners, raw honey and coconut sap. We discuss those in more detail in Chapter 8.

As for the artificial sweeteners on the list, they're questionable at best, toxic at worst, and not enough research has been done for us to safely condone any of them.

Sweeteners to avoid:

- Artificial sweeteners such as Aspartame, Sucralose, NutraSweet, and Splenda
- Brown sugar
- Corn syrup
- Glucose (dextrose)
- High-fructose corn syrup (also called corn sugar)
- Maltodextrin
- Maple syrup
- Molasses
- Raw sugar
- Refined honey (any honey that doesn't say "raw honey")
- Rice syrup
- Sugar alcohols (xylitol, mannitol, erythritol)
- Sugar cane or sugar cane juice
- White sugar

## Vegetable and Seed Oils

These include any oil that is hydrogenated, partially hydrogenated, fractionated, refined, or made from a legume or a grain. Even if it's one of the acceptable Paleo oils, like coconut or palm, if it's hydrogenated, fractionated, deodorized, bleached, or otherwise adulterated, don't eat it.

Oils to avoid:

- Canola oil
- Corn oil
- Cottonseed oil
- Margarine
- Palm kernel oil
- Peanut oil
- Safflower seed oil
- Soybean oil
- Sunflower seed oil
- Vegetable oil

**PALEO COMPASS**

Sunflower seeds are acceptable, but sunflower seed oil is unacceptable because the oil contains mostly omega-6 fatty acids. When it's consumed in large amounts (unlike sunflower seeds), it throws off the omega-6 to omega-3 ratio, promoting inflammation. It's also usually highly processed and heated. The same can be said for all the other oils except canola. The problem with canola is that it's usually highly processed and therefore highly oxidized by the time it hits the shelf. See "Canola Oil" later in this chapter.

## Fruit Juice

Unless it comes straight from a juicer, fruit juices are usually loaded with extra sugar, pasteurized (stripped of nutrients), and stripped of any fiber. The fiber in whole fruit buffers the high glycemic response to the sugary juice. There are beneficial nutrients in juice, especially when it's freshly juiced, but the blood sugar spike just doesn't warrant consuming it regularly.

## Soft Drinks and Other Sugary Drinks

Soft drinks, "sports" drinks, and other beverages with added sugar, artificial sweeteners, and additives are an unnecessary (even for most athletes) addition to the Western diet.

## Refined, Iodized Salt

Use unrefined sea salt instead of refined, iodized salt. Salt, or the flavorful sodium in it, has always been present in seafood, and was procured from sea water and the ashes of burned grass by hunter-gatherers. Sea salt provides more trace minerals than refined, iodized salt, which often has corn products and other unnecessary ingredients added to it.

Refined salt is chemically treated to purify it and make it white. Table salt is also treated with several anticaking chemicals, some of which contain aluminum, which competes with calcium for absorption and may decrease bone density and has been linked with neurological disorders, among other things.

Table salt is iodized in order to help prevent goiter, but there's actually iodine in many whole foods. Seaweed like kelp has the most iodine in it. Other good sources include asparagus, cod, eggs, garlic, mushrooms, sea salt, shrimp, spinach, strawberries, summer squash, Swiss chard, and tuna.

# Is It Paleo or Not?

This chapter is meant to be a compass, guiding you through grocery stores, restaurants, and get-togethers. But the guidelines we've put forth are not absolutely definitive because over the years, with evolving research, the "rules" of Paleo have changed. There are foods whose "Paleoness" has been hotly debated, and we discuss some of them here.

## Canola Oil

Canola oil has a pretty good ratio of omega-6 to omega-3—about 2:1—which is why it was first lauded in the Paleo world by Dr. Loren Cordain, health and exercise science professor at Colorado State University and leading expert on the Paleolithic diet. However, he no longer advocates the use of canola oil, as he recently stated in his book, *The Paleo Diet* (see Appendix B).

Canola oil contains erucic acid, which has been shown to cause allergic reactions in people and impair heart function in rats. It's also usually highly processed and heated, rendering its fragile omega-3s and omega-6s *oxidized*. Oxidized fats are implicated in inflammation and heart disease.

> **DEFINITION**
>
> Oils and fats become **oxidized** when they are exposed to too much heat, light, and air the same way that metal rusts when it's oxidized. The less stable the fatty acids are (omega-3s and -6s are less stable than monounsaturated, which are less stable than saturated), the more easily they oxidize. More information on this can be found in Chapter 4.

It's best to stay away from this potentially hazardous oil, but especially when it's used in restaurants, where the hydrogenated or otherwise chemically treated versions are usually used.

## Flaxseed Oil

Flax was originally suggested as a cooking and salad oil for Paleo eaters. However, we now know that because it's made of mostly unstable polyunsaturated fats, it can oxidize very easily when it's exposed to heat. That means you should never cook with the oil. If you use it at all, pour it over salads unheated and keep it in a cool, dark place to avoid oxidation and throw it out after six months of opening it. Some people take flax oil to supplement their omega-3s. While it does contain many omega-3 fatty acids, they're in the form of alpha linoleic acid (ALA). ALA is inefficiently converted into the anti-inflammatory omega-3s (EPA and DHA) that your body can use. EPA and DHA are found in fish oil, so you're better off getting your omega-3s from animal foods and not messing with such unstable oils like flax.

## Agave Nectar

Agave nectar is supposedly a natural sweetener, but it's often highly heated and chemically treated by the time it hits the shelves. It's also higher in fructose than other sweeteners, which has been shown to have a large effect on diabetes and weight gain. In general, stick with the other Paleo sweeteners.

## Vinegar

Vinegar is found in salad dressings and other packaged foods that would otherwise be Paleo, so people are often curious about it. It may have negative effects on people with autoimmune disorders. However, not everyone has autoimmune disorders and there are many beneficial effects of fermented foods. Ironically, both the negative and positive effects stem from some digestive function. We suggest you take note of how vinegar affects your digestion, and make your decision based on that. Don't make it a daily part of your diet.

**PALEO COMPASS**

The best vinegars to use are apple cider vinegar and balsamic, which don't contain gluten or non-Paleo ingredients. Malt vinegar is not technically Paleo because it's made of rye and is not distilled to remove the gluten. If you don't want to eat vinegar, freshly squeezed lemon and lime work very well as substitutes.

## Alcohol

There are healthy hunter-gatherer societies that imbibe alcoholic beverages, one being the Maasai of Africa. As we all know, though, alcohol consumption can be bad for our health, causing blood sugar imbalances and contributing to insulin resistance and diabetes, not to mention the dreaded "beer belly."

Speaking of which, beer is a favorite among many, and it's generally made with gluten grains. That terrible hangover and flushed skin may be due to the gluten in your favorite beer. We suggest you stop drinking alcohol for the first month on the diet, then add it back in to see how it affects you.

## Chocolate

As long as it's dark (more than 50 percent cocoa), we say eat it every once in a while. Chocolate is one of life's antioxidant rich delights, and even though it contains some sugar, it's okay to treat yourself once in a while. Its bliss-eliciting chemical properties may take you down a slippery slope, though, so keep it under control. Chocolate once a week seems reasonable.

## Coffee and Caffeinated Beverages

Although there are hunter-gatherer people who chew on stimulant leaves like betel or kava, coffee and "energy" drinks are on a different level. The caffeine in those drinks increases not only your blood pressure and heart rate, but your blood sugar levels, too. People become dependent on coffee to suppress their appetite and keep them awake, and it can really mess with cortisol levels (and therefore increase inflammation and belly fat). Food is a much better option for regulating your blood sugar.

Enjoy coffee on occasion because it tastes good—not as an addiction four times a day because it keeps you awake and regular. We suggest you remove coffee and other caffeinated drinks from your diet for the first month, and experiment with drinking caffeine after that. After a month away from it, you'll really be able to tell how it affects you.

## Potatoes and Other Nightshades

Potatoes are part of the nightshade family (tomato, potato, eggplant, bell pepper, paprika, chili peppers, and tobacco), which is a group of foods that can negatively affect people with autoimmune disorders. Nightshades have anecdotally caused joint pain in people who don't even have autoimmune disorders. Potatoes also contain the antinutrients saponins and solanine, which may cause digestive issues and potentially increase leaky gut.

If you have joint pain or an autoimmune disorder, don't eat any nightshades for the first month on the diet. Then put one of the nightshade foods back in your diet every week to see if they cause any symptoms. If you find that potatoes don't negatively affect you and you're an active person who tolerates moderate amounts of high glycemic foods, go ahead and eat them in moderation. You're much better off eating potatoes than grains or legumes.

## Dairy

As we've discussed, dairy is more appropriate for some people than for others. Many people just can't tolerate it: they're either lactose intolerant (even with the help of the lactase in raw dairy) or allergic to the casein (protein) in it, both of which can cause digestive problems, skin issues, joint aches, foggy thinking, vaginal yeast infections, and more.

Some studies on dairy have shown that casein induces the growth of cancer cells. Other studies have concluded that conjugated linoleic acid (CLA), which is found in the fat of milk, is a potent cancer fighter. That's why, if you're going to eat dairy, make it full-fat dairy, like cream, butter, or ghee (clarified butter). You need that fat to balance out the casein.

Fermented or aged milk products, like aged cheese, yogurt, kefir, buttermilk, and sour cream, are good choices because the fermentation process gets rid of much of the lactose in the milk. Since so many people are lactose intolerant, this allows them to eat dairy with less of a problem. Dairy from grass-fed animals is also a good choice because the grasses impart more vitamins, minerals, and CLA—that cancer fighter—to the milk. Most grass-fed dairy is also organic, which means no pesticides or added hormones are in the milk.

Also, look for raw dairy products, because the pasteurization process rids the milk of crucial enzymes that help us digest the milk and assimilate its nutrients. The homogenization process also places a tremendous amount of pressure and heat on the milk, changing the size and structure of the fat globules. The fat globules end up having whey and casein—proteins—in or on their walls. Studies have shown that those protein-laden fat globules can increase milk's ability to cause allergic reactions.

**PALEO COMPASS**

Raw dairy has a reputation for being dangerous because of harmful bacteria that can live in it. In fact, if you get your raw dairy from a small, well-managed local farm, there is little chance that it will be contaminated. Most producers test their milk regularly for any harmful substances and should be willing to show you the results of those tests. To find raw milk in your area, go to realmilk.com.

After a lifetime of eating foods that wreak havoc on our digestive systems, we're more prone to being affected negatively by dairy, since it's difficult to digest to begin with. The take-home of all this is that if you're going to consume dairy, it's absolutely best that you eat fermented, full-fat, raw milk products that came from grass-fed animals—and preferably only after a hard workout, when your cells are primed for the high insulin spike that dairy causes, which helps shuttle fuel into your cells.

## The Least You Need to Know

- Meat, fish, eggs, veggies, nuts, and seeds should make up the bulk of your Paleolithic diet.
- You can still enjoy chocolate, coffee, alcohol, and other foods—there's no reason to deny yourself those pleasures of life as long as you consume them in moderation.
- To reach your health goals, try to avoid grains, beans, vegetable oils, refined sugars, and pasteurized dairy products.
- Know the facts behind the debated Paleo foods so you can make an informed choice to eat them or not.

# Breaking Down the Diet

## In This Chapter

- A sample daily menu
- Macronutrient breakdown: protein, fat, and carbs
- The truth about high-protein diets, cholesterol, and saturated fat
- What the latest research says
- Paleo testimonials

Hopefully by now this is all sounding like a good direction to take your diet and your life. You can see how this all makes sense, and that the foods in the Paleolithic diet (listed in Chapter 3) actually look delicious and satisfying! However, if you are used to grains filling up a good portion of your plate and sugar dominating your snacks, what do you eat? We discuss a sample menu in this chapter and tell you how the protein, fat, and carbs should stack up on your plate.

After years of eating a Western diet, the thought of embracing meat and eggs—things you've been conditioned to avoid—is probably a little intimidating. We'll take on some common misconceptions about those very important foods so you can enjoy them without guilt or fear.

## Sample Menu

Following is a sample of one day in the life of a 35-year-old woman who weighs 130 pounds, who we'll call Lucy. She's not trying to lose weight, and she works out three times a week jogging, doing yoga, and other exercise. She needs about 2,000 calories per day to maintain her weight.

## Lucy's Typical Diet

|  | Calories | Carbs(g) | Fat(g) | Protein(g) |
|---|---|---|---|---|
| *Breakfast* | | | | |
| Roasted Pepper and Sausage Omelet (2 eggs) | 378 | 6 | 30 | 30 |
| 1 cup Sweet Potato Hash | 142 | 22 | 6 | 3 |
| *Lunch* | | | | |
| Cilantro Turkey Burger (4 oz.) with guacamole | 333 | 2 | 18 | 30 |
| 2 cups raw spinach | 14 | 2 | 0 | 2 |
| 1 cup cantaloupe | 60 | 14 | 0 | 1 |
| *Snack* | | | | |
| 2 oz. beef jerky | 150 | 4 | 4 | 14 |
| 1 oz. almonds (23 nuts) | 164 | 6 | 14 | 6 |
| 10 strawberries and ½ cup blueberries | 102 | 23 | 0 | .5 |
| *Dinner* | | | | |
| 5 oz. wild salmon | 257 | 0 | 11 | 36 |
| 2 cups cauliflower and broccoli sauté | 199 | 15 | 16 | 6 |
| *Dessert* | | | | |
| Carrot Banana Muffin | 288 | 24 | 20 | 8 |
| **Totals** | **2,087** | **118** | **119** | **137** |
| Percentage of calories | | 23% | 51% | 26% |
| U.S. average | 2,154 | 280 | 79 | 81 |
| Percentage of calories | | 52% | 33% | 15% |

# Recommended Protein, Fat, and Carb Intake

The point of the Paleolithic diet is not to have you counting grams, calories, or ounces. In order for this to be a sustainable way of life, you can't be charting out your daily food consumption for the rest of your life. The ultimate goal is for you to have a good sense of how much food your particular body needs and what proportions of carbohydrates, fat, and protein work best for you. In the beginning, you might need some help getting on track, though, after so many years of eating way too many carbs and probably not enough protein. Here are some guidelines to help get you started.

> **PALEO COMPASS**
>
> The intake of carbs, protein, and fat sometimes greatly differed among hunter-gatherer societies. For example, the islander Kitavans eat a diet that's about 70 percent carbohydrates, 20 percent fat, and 10 percent protein, while the native Inuits ate exclusively fatty, protein-rich animal foods for much of the year, at about 80 percent fat and 20 percent protein and virtually no carbohydrates. Those ratios aren't the norm, though: most other hunter-gatherer societies fell somewhere between those two cultures.

Given the information we have about what hunter-gatherers ate and the fact that most people in the Western world are overweight, we recommend you stay within the following *macronutrient* ranges. Staying near the low end of the carbohydrate range will promote weight loss, while the upper end will help an avid endurance athlete perform well.

- Carbohydrates: 10 to 40 percent

- Fat: 30 to 70 percent

- Protein: 20 to 35 percent

To put that into perspective, the average Western diet consists of about:

- Carbohydrates: 52 percent

- Fat: 33 percent

- Protein: 15 percent

**DEFINITION**

A **macronutrient** is any one of the three classes of chemical compounds we consume in the largest quantities, and from which we derive calories: carbohydrates, fats, and proteins.

It's clear that the Western diet provides less protein and more carbohydrates than that of the hunter-gatherers. But even though the percentage of fat is within the Paleolithic diet guidelines, the *quality* of fat is much different: vegetable oil accounts for about 80 percent of the fat in the Western diet, as opposed to the easily harvested fats found in animal foods and plants like nuts and coconuts. Let's put all these percentages into real life amounts for you now.

## Protein

If you're not into percentages, another useful way of figuring out how much protein you need is by looking at it in terms of grams. You should eat anywhere from 0.7 to 1 gram of protein per pound of *lean* body weight. If you're an athlete, aim for the upper end of that. If you weigh 150 pounds and have 25 percent body fat, that means 112.5 pounds of your weight is lean body mass. You'd want to eat anywhere from 79 (112.5 × .7) to 112.5 (112.5 × 1) grams of protein on average every day. Some days may be higher or lower than others, just like Lucy is having a high-protein day in the sample menu. On a different day her protein intake may be lower, so this high day makes up for that.

If you don't know what your lean body mass is, you can easily find out by going to a gym and asking a trainer to measure your body fat with calipers. There are more precise ways of measuring, but this is usually quick and inexpensive. It's also a good reason to go into the gym and stay for a workout!

To figure out exactly what the right amount of protein looks like on your own daily menu, refer to the protein content of some common foods in Appendix D. Lucy's sample menu gives you a good idea of what that looks like for a fairly active 130-pound woman eating 2,000 calories per day. Notice she had around 4 ounces of meat per meal, or around two eggs accompanied by a few ounces of meat. On lighter protein days, maybe Lucy would just have the eggs and no meat with them, or she'd have a less protein-dense snack.

If you're wondering about using protein powders, we don't suggest you rely too heavily on them. Meat, fish, and eggs are dense sources of protein. Powders are unnecessary, unless you're a large-bodied, serious athlete and you just can't stomach as much food as it would take to get you to your protein goals. Most protein powder options are non-Paleo, or debatably Paleo at best: they contain whey (dairy), soy, rice, pea, and other ingredients. The only one that would be truly Paleo is egg white protein, but it's highly processed to get it to its powder form. Plus, eggs are cheap—just eat those!

**NUTRITION FACT**

There is a physiological upper limit to protein intake: around 200 to 300 grams per day. If you eat more than about 40 percent of your calories as protein, you risk suffering from "rabbit starvation." Fur trappers in the 1800s who subsisted for too long on very lean meat (like from small animals such as rabbits) eventually experienced an intense craving for fat before they ended up dying of malnutrition.

## Fat

Fat can be efficiently transformed into glucose to be used by your body for energy. So can protein, but it's better to use the protein you eat for things like repairing muscle and tissue, and fortifying your immune system. Fat is important when you're eating this relatively low-carbohydrate diet: if you don't have the quick source of glucose that an abundance of sugar, grains, and beans supplies, you need to fuel yourself with plenty of fat.

The *kind* of fat you eat is incredibly important, and if you're following the food guidelines in this book, you should be on the right track. The type and quality of fats from meat vary depending on what kind of animal it is and what that animal ate. For instance, beef is fattier than chicken, and beef from a grass-fed cow is generally going to be less fatty than from a grain-fed cow. The amount of fat isn't quite as important as the kind of fat, though. Grass-fed animals provide a lot more conjugated linoleic acid (CLA), which is an anti-inflammatory, good fat. Grain-fed animals contain more omega-6 fatty acids, which we know are pro-inflammatory.

In 2002, Loren Cordain and several others published a study analyzing the diets of 229 modern, healthy hunter-gatherer groups in the *Journal of the American Nutraceutical Association*. Most of the groups derived between 56 and 65 percent of their calories from animal foods when possible. That's quite a large percentage of foods that are chock full of the fats you've been told to shun your whole life.

On average, the 229 hunter-gatherer groups ate anywhere from 30 to 60 percent of their total calories in fat, which is within the range we suggest you aim for. Knowing that that's an average, and that many cultures did very well on more fat than even 60 percent, some Paleo experts advise people to eat up to 80 percent fat. We don't see a problem with that, but some people would just rather not eat that much fat. You may have a twinge of skepticism about eating that much fat, but in the next section we hope to ease your mind a bit by busting some saturated fat and cholesterol myths.

All those percentages don't mean much to most people, though, so let's break this down into simpler terms. In the sample menu we presented earlier, Lucy is eating a 2,000-calorie diet. Fat is 9 calories per gram, so she's aiming for between 67 (30 percent total calories) and 156 (70 percent total calories) grams of fat per day. (See Appendix D for the fat content of some common foods.) This is quite a bit more than the USDA's recommended daily intake, but without those empty starches in your diet, you'll need this for energy. Only now it will be sustainable energy instead of the quickly rising and quickly plummeting energy that sugar and grains provide. The sample menu will give you a good idea of how that looks on Lucy's plate.

## Carbohydrates

Carbohydrates are the one macronutrient that we don't technically need in order to survive. The brain needs about 140 grams of glucose every day (and that estimate is high), but your body doesn't need dietary carbohydrates to make that: it can create it out of protein and fat.

The fact that we don't need carbohydrates makes sense if you think about what many of our ancestors ate: nothing but meat and fat during the winter when there were no vegetables or fruits to be found. We evolved to use fat and protein as fuel—not to constantly replenish our glucose levels with carbohydrates every few hours. If we needed as many carbs as the food pyramid says we do, we never would have survived the long, harsh winters over the 2.5 million+ years of our evolution.

As you start to use fat more efficiently for energy, instead of an overload of unnecessary carbs, your dependence on carbs starts to diminish. And your insulin and blood sugar levels begin to do the same.

The recommended amount of carbohydrates on this diet is between 20 and 40 percent to maintain your weight, but if you wanted to go below the 20 percent to lose weight more rapidly, you could, and many Paleo people do. If you need more concrete numbers, Mark Sisson, a prominent author and authority in the Paleo (or as he calls it, "primal") community of marksdailyapple.com created some guidelines that we agree with. If you're not an endurance athlete, stay between about 100 and 150 grams of carbs every day to maintain your weight. Lucy's sample menu will give you an idea of what your meals might look like when you're maintaining your weight. At 116 grams, she's within that 100- to 150-gram range. If you're actively trying to lose weight, stay between 50 and 100 grams, and if you're *really* die-hard about losing weight, you can try to go under that, but it's not advisable if you're working out a lot. On a 2,000-calorie diet, 20 percent of total calories equals 100 grams of carbs and the high end at 40 percent would be 200 grams. Two hundred grams and above would be reserved for serious endurance athletes. We talk more about athletes' specific needs in Chapter 6.

# Myths About Protein, Cholesterol, and Fat

If you're a normal Western person who has heard any negative press on high-protein diets, fat, or eggs, you might be wondering if the Paleolithic diet is going to make your arteries clog, your kidneys fail, and your bones fall prey to acid overload. Let's take a closer look at some of the myths.

## The Protein Fallacy

For the last 50 years, negativity and misconceptions have surrounded the topic of high-protein diets. But before we dispel some of that, we need to define what *exactly* a high-protein diet is. Sometimes it's defined as around 30 percent of the diet. In his protein debate with T. Colin Campbell (author of *The China Study*), Loren Cordain states that "high protein" is 20 to 29 percent of the daily calories and "very high protein" is 30 to 39 percent of daily calories. That means if you were eating 2,000 calories per day on a standard Western diet, you'd be getting around 75 grams of protein per day. On a high-protein diet, it would be anywhere from 100 to 145 grams per day. And a very high-protein diet would provide 150 to 195 grams. (Remember, Lucy's sample menu contains 133 grams, for reference, which she got primarily from meat, fish, and eggs.)

### Minimum Protein Requirement

The USDA states that a 19- to 70-year-old man can survive, and perhaps even thrive, on 56 grams of protein a day. For a man eating 2,000 calories per day, that's only about 11 percent of his diet. That's about the same percentage that T. Colin Campbell advocates, along with other vegan proponents: 10 percent protein.

### Maximum Protein Intake

When you eat too much protein, your liver can no longer make urea (a waste product from protein that's excreted in the urine), and ammonia leaks into your bloodstream, eventually causing death. We've mentioned this before: it's called rabbit starvation, and it happens when you eat too much lean protein with not enough fat or carbohydrates to buffer it.

The liver's upper limit of protein intake is about 200 to 300 grams per day, or about 35 to 40 percent of caloric intake. The Paleolithic diet, however, doesn't advocate eating more than 35 percent protein. It's even rare for hunter-gatherer groups to eat more protein than that because they know the consequences. So yes, the Paleolithic diet has a *higher* protein percentage than the 15 percent in the typical Western diet, but it's well within the safe limits of what your body can handle.

### High Protein and Your Kidneys

What about the effect of a high-protein diet on the kidneys? There is some alarming research on the effect of high-protein diets on the kidneys, but the truth is the subjects of those studies *already had kidney disease* when they started the high-protein diets. All the research on people with normally functioning kidneys concludes that they do just fine on high-protein diets, as they have for 2.5 million years.

As the National Kidney Foundation states, "Diabetes is the leading cause of kidney disease"—not a high-protein diet. So if you're worried about your kidneys, it looks like the typical, high-glycemic Western diet is more dangerous than a healthy dose of protein.

## Cholesterol and Saturated Fat Fables

Both cholesterol and saturated fat have pretty terrible reputations in the Western world, and for outdated and unsupported reasons. The change from healthy animal fats to wrecked, omega-6-laden oils is one of the greatest mistakes we made in the last century.

### Cholesterol

For the last 50 years, the media has overwhelmed us with the heart health merits of a low-cholesterol diet. "Meat and eggs will clog your arteries," we're warned. "Keep it under 300 mg of cholesterol a day," they caution. The truth is clear, though: even the researchers who started the cholesterol craze no longer believe that dietary cholesterol has anything to do with the risk of heart disease.

Ancel Keys (a.k.a. "Monsieur Cholesterol") was partly responsible for proliferating the cholesterol myths in the early 1900s. Even he later discounted the idea that dietary cholesterol causes heart disease, saying "It is now clear that dietary cholesterol per se, which is contained in almost all foods of animal origin, has little or no effect on the serum cholesterol concentration in man."

**PALEO COMPASS**

Early studies that kicked off the cholesterol scare showed that if you fed rabbits a high-cholesterol diet, it caused atherosclerosis, or plaque build-up on the walls of their arteries. That would be terrible news if rabbits' dietary needs were anything like our own. However, they're specifically designed to eat mostly plants, unlike humans. It's like feeding pork chops to a cow and being surprised when it gets sick.

In 1970, the Framingham Heart Study, one of the largest and most influential studies on heart health done to date, concluded that dietary cholesterol had absolutely no effect on serum cholesterol levels (the cholesterol levels your doctor tests). In 1971, one of the researchers from that study, George Mann, went on to examine the primitive Maasai people in Africa, who eat mainly raw cow's milk and meat. Their overwhelming lack of heart disease led Mann to conclude that "The diet-heart hypothesis has been repeatedly shown to be wrong, and yet, for complicated reasons or pride, profit and prejudice, the hypothesis continues to be exploited by scientists, fund-raising enterprises, food companies, and even governmental agencies. The public is being deceived by the greatest health scam of the century."

**Why All the Cholesterol Fuss?**

Despite the fact that even the originators of the cholesterol hype are now abandoning their initial claims, the general public, food manufacturers, and medical professionals still clutch to their fear of eating eggs and meat. The theory goes like this: heart disease is correlated with high levels of cholesterol in the blood, so lowering dietary cholesterol should decrease the chances of developing heart disease. In reality, that over-simplified theory is severely flawed. Here's why.

Cholesterol is such a necessary component of the human body that we produce anywhere from 1,000 to 1,400 milligrams of the stuff on our own every day (a lot more than the 180 milligrams you'll find in an egg). We need it to make hormones, bile, every one of your cell membranes, skin, and brain cells, among other things. When we eat dietary cholesterol from animal foods, our body uses what it needs and excretes the rest.

Aside from a small percentage of people, our intelligent bodies regulate cholesterol by producing less of it in response to eating it. A 2006 study published in *Current Opinion in Clinical Nutrition and Metabolic Care* clearly showed that 70 percent of the population's blood cholesterol levels were unaffected by eating eggs, while 30 percent had an increase in both *low-density lipoprotein* (*LDL*) and *high-density lipoprotein* (*HDL*).

> **DEFINITION**
>
> **Low-density lipoprotein (LDL)** or "bad" cholesterol is a combination of protein, triglycerides, and cholesterol that transports cholesterol from the liver to other cells of the body for use. **High-density lipoprotein (HDL)** or "good" cholesterol is a combination of protein, triglycerides, and cholesterol that transports cholesterol from cells of the body back to the liver.

An increase in LDL and HDL is not necessarily a bad thing. LDL was once thought to be the "bad" cholesterol, but further investigation has shown that a few other things are more important risk factors for heart disease:

- Small, dense LDL particles—we'll call it the "bad LDL"—and specifically those that are oxidized, may be one of the real culprits of heart disease. The small, dense, bad LDL is more susceptible to oxidation than the more stable, large, buoyant LDL, which we'll call the "good LDL." Good LDL is the kind of LDL that increases in some people when they eat dietary cholesterol and saturated fat. On the other hand, bad LDL can increase when you eat a carbohydrate-rich Western diet. Translation: cholesterol and saturated fat are fine; excess simple carbohydrates are not.

- Excess fructose (refined sugar, high-fructose corn syrup, etc.), lack of exercise, smoking, excessive alcohol, high blood sugar from eating too many simple carbs, and omega-6 fatty acids can all cause oxidation of bad LDL.

- Oxidized LDL is associated with "plaque ruptures," which happen when plaque build-up breaks off artery walls and causes strokes and heart attacks. Plaque is made up of a disproportionate amount of linoleic acid, an omega-6 fatty acid found in "heart-healthy" vegetable oils. They've found that the amount of linoleic acid in the bloodstream is determined by how much of it you eat.

- Another contributing factor to heart disease is damage to the arterial walls caused by a high-carbohydrate diet, smoking, stress, high omega-6 to omega-3 ratio, and trans fats.

## A Faulty Theory

Remember that the "lipid theory," as it's known, goes like this: heart disease is caused by high levels of cholesterol in the blood, so lowering dietary cholesterol should decrease the chances of developing heart disease. We now know that:

- Dietary cholesterol has little to no effect on blood cholesterol levels.

- The effect dietary cholesterol may have on blood cholesterol does not necessarily lead to heart disease. In fact, high levels of blood cholesterol aren't, and have never been, a reliable predictor of heart disease.

- The lifestyle and dietary habits that actually contribute to heart disease are the same that lead to obesity and diabetes: too many omega-6 fatty acids, which help promote chronic inflammation of the arterial walls; high glycemic foods like sugar and refined grains; and not exercising.

The original theory was wrong in every way, and even the original propagators of that theory know it. Your arteries don't get clogged by animal fat. That's just not the way it works.

 **DAMAGE CONTROL**

According to the Centers for Disease Control and Prevention (CDC), a whopping 54 percent of adults over 20 used cholesterol-lowering drugs in 2006 in the United States. Even with all the statin drugs and other cholesterol-lowering pharmaceuticals out there, heart disease is still the leading cause of death in America and the entire world.

## Saturated Fat

This brings us to that evil substance, saturated fat. Or, at least that's what we're supposed to think of it. Saturated fat can, in fact, raise LDL levels, but it raises the *good* LDL we talked about before, which doesn't increase the incidence of heart disease. In fact, a paper by Siri-Tarino et al., published in 2010 in the *American Journal of Clinical Nutrition*, reviewed 21 studies, including 347,747 subjects, and concluded, "There is no significant evidence for concluding that dietary saturated fat is associated with an increased risk of CHD or CVD [heart disease]." But before scientists, even scientists who endorsed the Paleolithic diet, were aware of the distinction between the different kinds of LDL, they demonized saturated fat, including plant sources like coconut oil and palm oil.

Coconut oil or palm oil is actually a great source of medium-chain triglycerides (MCTs), a type of saturated fat that can be used very quickly as energy in the body. In many studies, MCTs have been shown to help people lose weight. One of the fatty acids in coconut oil, lauric acid, is a powerful antiviral and can also increase HDL, the "good" cholesterol in your body. So much for coconut oil's bad reputation!

## Clearing Up Some Paleo Confusion

In his first book, *The Paleo Diet* (see Appendix B), Loren Cordain decried saturated fat as a heart disease promoter. He urged people to either eat very lean cuts of meat that were mostly protein, or to eat grass-fed animals that have a lower saturated fat content. In light of the new research on the distinction between the different kinds of LDL and the importance of oxidation, this statement was made on Cordain's website (thepaleodiet.blogspot.com) in 2010: "The bottom line is that we do not recommend cutting down saturated fatty acid intake but rather decrease high-glycemic load foods, vegetable oils, refined sugars, grains, legumes and dairy."

It's important to note that eating Western foods *along with* eating a lot of fatty animal foods may increase your chances of creating oxidized LDL, and therefore heart disease, because the saturated fat increases LDL and the Western diet oxidizes it. When looking at the arteries of the frozen remains of ancient Alaskan Inuit people and recent autopsies of the modern African Masai, researchers found they did, in fact, have atherosclerosis, or plaque build-up in their arterial walls. However, there was no sign of any heart attacks or stroke, and no other record of them. The researchers believe that without the underlying inflammation and oxidation caused by Western foods, the plaque doesn't break off to cause heart attacks or strokes. This is yet another reason to eat a Paleolithic diet.

## What This Means for Your Diet

Paleo experts are all for wild, grass-fed animal meat and fat. In fact, we want you to eat the fat, the marrow, the meat, and the organs of animals just like our ancestors did. There are different nutrients in each part of the animal that you can benefit from. However, some meat and eggs are better than others. Problems with animal foods can occur when the animals are fed grains that cause them to gain excessive weight and have digestive distress and inflammation. They accumulate omega-6s just like we do from food, and those fatty acids end up in the meat we eat.

The USDA and Clemson University reported in 2009 that grass-fed beef was better for people in the following ways:

- Higher in beta-carotene (vitamin A precursor)
- Higher in vitamin E

- Higher in the B vitamins thiamin and riboflavin

- Higher in calcium, magnesium, and potassium

- Higher in total omega-3s

- A healthier ratio of omega-6 to omega-3 fatty acids (1.65 versus 4.84)

- Higher in conjugated linoleic acid (CLA), a potential cancer fighter

- Higher in vaccenic acid, which can be transformed into CLA

To put this into plain English, find the cleanest sources of meat, fish, and eggs possible. Look for meat that's wild or grass-fed. Then, knowing you're getting the nutrient profile closest to that we evolved eating, you can eat those foods without concern. Eat your beloved bacon. Feel free to eat the chicken skin and liver. Cook with meat drippings, and don't trim the fat off your meat if you don't want to. And don't forget to boil those bones to harvest the precious, fatty marrow.

All of those things sound almost sinful (but probably delicious) to the average American, and not many diet books have dared to go here before, but that's why the rest of the diets aren't working. We naturally need fat to feel satiated so we don't overeat and crave sugar, and animal fat is the best, most finger-lickin' good place to get it.

We highly suggest you eat only grass-fed, pasture-raised, or wild animal foods, but even if you're eating grain-fed animal foods, it's better than eating grains, refined carbs, and vegetable oils. If you do eat grain-fed, which is most of the stuff that's sold in conventional grocery stores, you will want to trim off the extra fat to avoid the omega-6s stored in it.

In short, you can feel confident that animal foods are what you're supposed to be eating, and what your ancestors sought out the most.

# Modern Paleo Studies: Does It Really Work?

We can talk all we want about how our Paleolithic ancestors and modern hunter-gatherer groups ate this way and enjoyed incredible health, but you probably want some modern research to back it up. It worked for them, but will it work for you? And how long did these people really live? Wasn't it only about 30 years? So let's look at some of the data. (We'll only be able to touch on this, there's plenty more research available if you start looking.)

## Kicking Diabetes in the Outback

One of the earlier controlled studies on eating Paleo was published in *Diabetes* in 1984, and conducted in Australia. Ten Aboriginal men spent the first part of their lives as hunter-gatherers, but ended up living in rural Australia, eating a Western diet. Predictably, they were all overweight with type 2 diabetes. They were asked to go back into the Outback and live as they had, eating only what they could hunt and gather: kangaroos, birds, crocodiles, turtles, shellfish, crayfish, yams, figs, and honey. After seven weeks, the average weight loss was 16.5 pounds. Blood cholesterol dropped by 12 percent and triglycerides by an astounding 72 percent. Their diabetes disappeared, as their insulin and glucose levels became normal.

## Paleo Beats Out Diabetes Diet

In a 2009 study, Dr. Staffan Lindeberg (known for his work with the primitive Kitavan society) compared the effectiveness of a Paleolithic diet versus the commonly recommended diabetes diet on 13 patients with type 2 diabetes. The diabetes diet was low-fat, low-meat, high-carb, and included whole grains, fruits, vegetable oils, vegetables, and dairy. The Paleolithic diet had better results for weight loss, blood pressure, waist size, triglycerides, HDL cholesterol (the good cholesterol), glucose levels, and hemoglobin A1c (a long-term marker for blood glucose levels).

## High Protein Keeps Weight Off

In 2010 a study published in the *New England Journal of Medicine* showed that a high-protein, low glycemic diet most effectively kept weight off of 773 subjects over 6 months.

In the same year a study of 827 overweight and obese children found that the kids who were put on a high-carb, low-protein diet became significantly fatter over 6 months, while the children on a high-protein, low-carb diet significantly lost weight.

# Paleo Success Stories

The studies speak volumes, but here is a testimonial from Richard, a 58-year-old man on the Paleolithic diet, in case you still don't believe us:

*I started the Paleolithic diet in mid-December 2010 with the intent of losing some weight and improving my overall health. I lost 25 pounds but got other benefits I never anticipated. First, I used to take antacids every day, starting in my mid-20s and developed acid reflux over the last few years. A few weeks after I started eating Paleo, I stopped them completely. Now the only times I take antacids are when I cheat on the diet with bread and sugar on the same day, and not always.*

*Second, I suffered from sinus headaches every month or so that would last up to 3 days at a time. Since I started Paleo, I have only had one headache. I also had pain in my elbow due to an injury lifting weights, and every time I exercised it would hurt. Now there is no pain in that elbow at all. I attribute this to a decrease in inflammation.*

*Finally, my overall energy and focus have increased dramatically, even though I "cheat" on the diet once a week. I feel great, have maintained my target weight, and lost some ailments I previously attributed to aging. What a great diet!*

Here's what Mindy, a 31-year-old woman, has to say about the effect of Paleo on her rheumatoid arthritis:

*Getting diagnosed with severe rheumatoid arthritis (RA) when I was 25 was fairly terrifying. I did everything my doctors told me: took my medications; eliminated stress; kept my weight regular; and maintained an active lifestyle, including yoga. Thankfully I responded well to the lifestyle change. However, the medications were horrible; not only did they make me feel like a zombie, but they were extremely toxic and dangerous to my body, requiring constant trips to the doctor and labs to make sure I was okay. While I was open to switching my diet, I was very concerned about my long-term health; RA is progressive and degenerative, which means I'll always have it and it will only get worse over time. I thought diet couldn't possibly help with the magnitude of my disease.*

*A co-worker who has a different autoimmune disease happened to mention the Paleo diet in an email, and she said it had really helped her symptoms. At this point, I'd been on and off my medications for over 6 years and I was more open to seeing how diet might affect my health. I started the Paleo diet in December 2010 and have been going strong for nearly a year. Over the course of the year, I had to take a break from my medications because of getting pneumonia. When the pneumonia passed, my RA symptoms did not return. I waited a week to start taking my medications again and still no swelling in my fingers, no aching in my joints. Nothing.*

*I realized that maybe the diet was actually having a much deeper effect on my body and was filled with unbelievable hope. My grandmother had crippling RA and was never able to hold me, go on walks with me, or do anything but talk with me at her bedside. She was bedridden my whole life because of her RA. The idea that I might be able to be healthy without my medication was a dream beyond dreams; I didn't want to be that crippled woman unable to engage with her family and life. Every day I wake up and wonder if the symptoms will come back—and someday they might—but I feel tremendous. My body is as strong as it's ever been, and I feel as good as I have in years. I feel like I get to eat the richest, tastiest foods in the world and am proactively contributing to my own health in way that is immensely empowering. I plan to eat Paleo for the rest of my life, whether I have to take my medication again or not.*

## The Least You Need to Know

- It is easier than you think to eat healthy, delicious food that conforms to the Paleolithic diet.
- Compared with the Western diet, Paleo is higher in protein and fat and lower in carbohydrates.
- High-protein diets are good for most people, and the fats in meat and eggs don't cause heart disease: inflammatory Western foods do.
- Research shows that modern people eating Paleo overcame diabetes, lost weight (and kept it off), and improved their cholesterol levels.
- Real people are having amazing turnarounds in their weight and health by eating the Paleolithic diet.

# Implementing Paleo

If you've ever dieted—and it's statistically likely you have—you know that diets can be hard to stick with. The foods can be unsatisfying and tasteless, and you often end up hungry. Luckily, eating Paleo isn't necessarily a "diet" like you might be accustomed to: you'll feel full and satisfied by delicious, wholesome foods. However, there are some things you need to adjust to when eating Paleo.

In this part, we give you tips on implementing the diet and then actually sticking with it. You learn about "cheating" to make the diet sustainable, what to eat when you go to restaurants or travel, how to modify the diet as an athlete, and how to make food prep and cooking as simple as possible. We also go into the big question: can you afford to eat this way?

# Eating Paleo in a Non-Paleo World

## In This Chapter

- Getting your family on board
- Why it's okay to cheat once in a while
- Eating out and traveling
- Can a vegetarian eat Paleo?
- The kosher Paleolithic diet
- What about supplements?

While this diet does have some serious merits, you're definitely straying from the norm by taking it on. You're going to have to make your way through normal daily life, and possibly help guide your family, too.

You're not cave people eating from the fertile land anymore. You have children who go to grain-mongering schools. You have jobs that require travel to non-Paleo-friendly places, and you go on vacations where good food may be hard to come by. The soil around us has become depleted from poor farming practices. And besides all that, there are religions that keep people from eating particular foods. How do you navigate this Neolithic world while still eating Paleo? It's definitely possible, and in this chapter, we show you how.

## Raising a Paleo Family

Your friends are one thing—you can tell them about a diet and they can choose to take it on or not. But your spouse and kids? You live with them, and it's going to be a little difficult to cook and eat different meals than theirs every day. Plus, you have a vested interest in their health, and you probably want them to eat this way, too. It's time to consider whether or not you want to take this change family-wide or just do it on your own.

> **PALEO COMPASS**
>
> People wonder whether or not this diet is okay for children, and the answer is absolutely. If adults are supposed to eat this way, and should have been all along, then kids are lucky if they're exposed to the Paleolithic diet as early on as possible. When you're mulling over what it's worth to you to take away your kids' beloved granola bars, cereals, cookies, and sodas, ask yourself what it's worth to them. It could be everything.

Your kids might be healthy right now, but it doesn't mean that if they continue on the dietary path they're on they won't become overweight, tired, and sick as adults. It only takes time for extra weight to appear and digestive disorders to settle into their bodies. There's no reason to wait until they feel bad or gain weight to make changes in their diet. Why not put them on this diet while they're ahead of the game?

People fall into the trap of giving kids "kid" food because they think they won't eat anything else. But if all you make available to them (as our hunter-gatherer ancestors did) are healthy proteins and fats served up with colorful fruits and veggies, they'll dig in because they're hungry and it tastes good. Eventually, they'll figure out that these foods also give them more energy and make them feel better overall.

There are a few common concerns parents have about putting their kids on a Paleolithic diet. One is about not eating dairy to get the necessary calcium for growing bones. Another question is whether their kids will get the right fats for a developing brain. And lastly, parents wonder if their kids will get enough nutrients in general. We've covered these topics throughout the book, and almost everything we've said about adults also applies to children. You can rest assured they'll get all the nutrients they need eating Paleo. We do recommend you make sure they get a variety of vegetables and proteins, as a broader base of food gives them a broader base of vitamins and minerals.

Check out Appendix E for a comparison of nutrients in the Western diet compared to a Paleolithic diet. Chapter 2 has a section on calcium that applies to children as well. Remember that the countries that consume the most dairy have the worst bone health. Dairy isn't necessarily all it's cracked up to be.

Without all those antinutrients in grains and legumes, kids will absorb way more of the vitamins and minerals they consume. Plus, veggies and meat have always had more nutrients in them than pasteurized skim milk, pasta, and granola bars.

## Getting the Kids on Board

But how will you get your kids to start the diet in the first place? It depends on how old they are, but education is a must. If they're old enough to understand, tell them why you're doing this, and what benefits they will gain. There's no child who's too young for this diet. During the weaning process, all children begin eating blended foods, including meats, vegetables, and fruits, all of which are Paleo foods. The only difference is now you'll be saving them from pasteurized dairy, something that is quite often the culprit in children's eczema, asthma, and other ailments. And you'll be doing them a favor by not nurturing their sweet tooth and spiking their blood sugar with grains and sugar. Remember, this is how children were raised for all of history until relatively recently.

With the protein and healthy fat-filled breakfasts, they're likely to be able to concentrate better in school. All the meals and snacks create even blood sugar, so they're less apt to have meltdowns and tantrums. Balanced blood sugar makes for more natural sleep patterns, too. If your child is overweight or struggling with acne, this diet will help, if not fix the problem. And what about the teen boy wanting more muscle mass? He'll probably notice the changes quicker than he expects. Teen girls will appreciate clearer, healthier skin and better fitting jeans. The lack of sugar and other immune suppressing foods in the diet will make your kids come home with fewer colds, too.

After you tell them about all the good that can come from eating Paleo, be sure to let them in on the not so good things that can happen when you grow up eating a Western diet. You might have some daunting first-hand experience about it: weight gain, lethargy, digestive problems, heart disease, diabetes, etc. Let them know the truth and the importance of the diet might just get through to them.

## Eating at School, Camp, and Friends' Houses

What about eating away from home? You can only supervise what your kids eat to a certain extent. When they're at parties, camp, or even at school, they might have way more freedom with food. That's why it's so important to clearly explain the benefits of Paleo and the pitfalls of the Western diet. That way, when they're out making their own choices, they'll have a foundation of knowledge from which to act.

Of course, it would be great if kids never wanted to eat a piece of normal birthday cake again, but that's not realistic. It's not even realistic for adults. Let your kids indulge sometimes, as long as they're not allergic to the foods they're indulging in. If you're at a gathering and your kids are feeling left out because they can't have cake and cookies, just allow it to happen sometimes. Especially if you haven't brought a Paleo-friendly substitution for them.

That doesn't mean every weekend you let your kids binge on cake and cookies, rendering the whole weekend a rollercoaster of tantrums and mood swings. Be firm when you need to, stick to your guns and be prepared for situations like that. But when it happens, it happens.

When you can, make Grain-Free Chocolate Chip Cookies, Almond Macaroons, or Carrot Cake (recipes in Chapter 16), or at the very least buy some gluten- and dairy-free snacks to substitute for the conventional treats they'll be tempted by. Associating the diet with negative situations won't make them want to adhere to it when they're making choices for themselves later on, so do what you can to avoid that.

We know this is a lot more work for parents, who are probably tired and overworked to begin with. But we've all seen parents make all sorts of sacrifices for their children when they get sick, especially when they get really sick. So be proactive and do what you can to give them the best, healthiest future possible.

> **PALEO COMPASS**
>
> Many Paleo parents find that over time, their kids realize that when they eat non-Paleo foods, they don't feel so great. They end up steering clear of the stuff on their own. Be patient with the process and try not to freak out when everything isn't perfectly Paleo.

Here are a few more tips for successfully making the Paleo switch with your kids:

- Ask them to help out in the kitchen—get them involved!

- Remember that kids are actually better at knowing when they're full and hungry than you are. Don't get discouraged if your kids don't want to eat exactly when you want them to all the time. Let them eat when they're hungry—just always have good options available for them when they are.

- Get rid of the junk food in the house. Nobody needs unhealthy temptations, and the presence of junk food is a huge source of our cravings; out of sight, out of mind.

- Start the diet on your own for a few weeks to a month. Get to know the diet yourself so you can help your family enjoy it with some tried-and-tested recipes, such as those in Part 3.

- Have fun with it and don't stress out too much—it doesn't have to be perfect all at once (or ever)!

# It's Okay to Cheat Sometimes

You may have just taken from that last section that it's okay for your kids to "cheat" on the diet sometimes. So if your kids can "cheat," can you? Yes. Please do. The Paleolithic diet movement has become so prolific because people figure out what they need to do to keep it sustainable.

> **PALEO COMPASS**
>
> Considering about 45 million people every year in the United States go on diets, spending billions of dollars on magic bullet diet products, there's a good chance you've been on a diet before. There's also a good chance you've failed on that diet because it was too restrictive. It's up to you to find the balance between restrictive and healthily satisfying.

Whether or not we like it, we're all faced with food temptations every day. A good rule of thumb is to stay true to the diet at least 85 percent of the time. If there are three meals and one snack every day, that means up to four meals or snacks every week can be non-Paleo. However, there are some exceptions to that rule. Like the kids, if you have a known allergy or severe sensitivity to a food, don't eat it. Also, if you need to lose weight, eating close to 100 percent Paleo will make the process go much faster.

In the end, like most Paleo eaters, you'll probably find that the more you eat Western foods, the worse you feel, so the cheating will be guided by your symptoms. The Paleolithic diet, in its purest form, is incredibly nourishing. What *isn't* nourishing is stress, though, so if that bowl of refined semolina pasta is what's going to relieve your feelings of dietary deprivation once every few weeks, dig in. But as you learn to listen to your body, you'll know how it'll affect you when you do dig in, so be extra-attentive when you do cheat.

# Eating Out

Eating in your own home is much easier because you have control over every single ingredient. But almost nobody eats at home every single meal, every day of the week. Here are some suggestions for staying on the Paleo wagon even when you're at a restaurant.

The simplest and most prevalent option is the salad. Almost all restaurants have some type of salad, and we recommend asking for olive oil with lemon or vinegar for dressing. Don't be afraid to add extra meat or hard-boiled eggs to make sure you get enough protein. Most places also have avocados or guacamole, which is a great source of fat and will help you feel full, especially if you're used to getting a burger and a pile of fries. You can eat the avocado on the side or add it to your salad so you don't go home hungry.

Alternatively, order a meat or seafood entrée with vegetables. If pasta, bread, or rice is a main component of the meal, ask them to hold the starch and add more vegetables or protein. There may be a slight up-charge, but consider that a tax for being healthy. You may save that money later on when you need less health care. If they won't accommodate special requests, a baked potato or sweet potato with olive oil would be way better than the grain-based alternatives.

**PALEO COMPASS**

Do some internet sleuthing or make phone calls to find out which restaurants in your area, if any, serve pasture-raised animal products. And when you find one, ask the restaurant who else does as well. Most restaurants that value grass-fed meat will know the other places that do, too. It's becoming more and more common for restaurants to use local sources for their meat, and it's usually advertised on their websites if they do. Check your favorite restaurants out or explore new food venues to get the best animal products you can.

If there isn't a suitable salad, meat, or seafood entrée, start looking at the sandwiches. In a pinch you can always order a burger or chicken sandwich without the bun or bread. Ask for a salad instead of the vegetable oil laden fries or potato chips. You might end up with two plates—one for the burger or chicken with no bun and one for the salad. Just mix the two together and you have yourself a beef or chicken salad. Again, olive oil with vinegar or lemon makes a great dressing and most restaurants have those ingredients.

At Asian restaurants you can usually find just a seafood and veggie dish. Otherwise, consider ordering an entrée without the rice or pasta. That would be a bit difficult with things like fried rice or Pad Thai, but curry is delicious even without the rice. Just be careful not to order it too spicy because the rice is usually what tones down the heat.

Italian restaurants often offer meat or seafood and veggie entrées. Just inquire about the dairy content in everything. And try to keep your hands off that bread! We recommend you tell them right when you sit down to not bother bringing it, that way, it won't be staring at you while you're hungry and waiting for your entrée.

And Mexican restaurants? Steak and veggie fajitas without the corn tortillas and sour cream are a good option, and almost universally available. Yes, you'll be eating corn oil or some other variety of vegetable oil no doubt, but it's better than eating a sour cream slathered burrito encased in a flour tortilla the size of your torso.

# Traveling

You're going to eat out more when you're on vacation or away on business, but try not to make those times free-for-all feeding frenzies (especially if you travel a lot). It takes some preparation and know-how, but it is possible to eat well on the road, whether you're traveling by plane or by car.

Airports and airplanes are not the most Paleo-friendly places in the world. In fact, they're almost certain death for the diet. You're hungry and trapped, so you're forced to buy whatever's available to you, which almost always involves grains, sugar, and dairy. The solution is to plan ahead.

You can bring food through the security line and onto the plane. As long as it's not liquid, you're fine, but even then there are some exceptions. For instance, almond butter will be confiscated, but a sweet potato slathered in coconut milk will not. On the day of your trip, double or triple the size of your breakfast or lunch so you have leftovers for the plane ride. Store them in containers and put them in your carry-on with some fruit. Food will last a day without being refrigerated if it's not in direct sun, but you can always bring one of those icepacks along.

Also, most airport newsstands sell jerky, trail mix, and fruit. These are important tools to get you through in a pinch and last several days. The trail mix probably has M&Ms or something similar in there, but it's better than a bagel and cream cheese, so be your own hunter and gatherer and see what you can scavenge.

For longer plane trips, take a bit of time to make more of what you'll need. Make extra dinner the night before so you have leftovers, or bake a batch of Almond Muffins (recipe in Chapter 16) and bring a few wrapped in tinfoil. Pack a bag of homemade Paleo Trail Mix (recipe in Chapter 11) or beef jerky, or hard-boil some eggs and put them in a container. Or do all of the above. You may need to bring a larger carry-on than you normally would, and your neighbors on the plane might shoot you some strange (perhaps jealous) looks, but at least you won't be hungry and desperate. Also, while it's going to be low-quality meat, you can always get a burger without the bun from just about any fast-food place in any airport. It'll be better than the food they offer you on the plane.

Now you've got your food in transit squared away, but what about when you arrive at your destination? That depends on whether you'll be staying at a hotel, a house, or a tent, and for how long. If you're staying at a hotel for a short period of time, just be sure to have plenty of snacks. If your hotel room has a refrigerator, or you're staying at someone's house, you can bring all kinds of foods in your checked luggage: a batch of roasted chicken breasts, a pound of cooked burgers, almond butter and fruit, a bag of chopped veggies, an entire batch of almond flour blueberry muffins, etc. If you come prepared with food, you're going to be less likely to binge on non-Paleo foods at restaurants and your host's home. Plus, you can bring enough muffins or other goodies to share with your host as a gift. Who knows? Maybe the food you share will entice them to try eating Paleo.

**PALEO COMPASS**

If you're staying with someone in their home, bring crucial items you don't think they'll have, or be prepared to go to a good grocery store shortly after you arrive. Research the restaurants in the area so you have some Paleo-friendly ideas for your nights and days out.

If you're going to be sightseeing, spending long hours away from the hotel or house, stick high-calorie snacks in your backpack or purse. Think trail mix and beef jerky. The last thing you want to do is get so hungry that you stop at the first fast-food restaurant you see and order the most super-sized, non-Paleo items on the menu.

And if you're at a conference or typical business trip, most places have bagels, fruit, pastries, and yogurt for snacks and breakfasts. This can be really tough if you're not prepared. Most hotels will know where you can get a quick breakfast burrito nearby, and just give yourself a bit of extra time with a fork to eat the guts and throw away the tortilla. They're quick, cheap, and the eggs and sausage can keep you satisfied until you get your lunch break. Just remember to ask for it without cheese and maybe double meat if you can.

# Paleo and Vegetarianism

Some people don't love the taste of meat, or have been vegetarians for so long that they can't fathom eating meat regularly. It's possible to eat a nutritious Paleolithic diet and not eat a lot of meat. If you're willing to eat plenty of eggs and fish, along with nuts, fruits, and veggies, you'll be able to get enough protein. But if you're unwilling to eat any meat, fish, or eggs, you probably won't see as many benefits as you would otherwise. If you have questions or concerns, check with a holistic health practitioner or nutritionist.

While some hunter-gatherer groups, like the Kitavans, do quite well with very little meat, fish, or eggs in their diets, they have the advantage of not having eaten processed, refined, very high glycemic and low-nutrient foods their whole lives, as many Westerners have. That means their blood sugar and inflammation levels are much healthier. You, on the other hand, probably need plenty of protein to help restore your blood sugar to normal levels and combat chronic inflammation. Consider eating more animal protein than you might be used to, for the sake of your health.

# Keeping Kosher While Eating Paleo

Eating kosher while trying to maintain a Paleolithic diet and lifestyle should pose only one major challenge: sourcing kosher animal products. The only kosher guideline that truly affects the diet is the selection of animal products you can eat. And that should only be an issue if you're following a meal plan, such as the one we've laid out in this book (see Chapter 18).

For instance, if a recipe calls for pork loin, you can always change it to any kosher meat. Chicken is often a good substitute for pork. As for shellfish, they can be substituted with any kosher seafood, or any meat for that matter.

Many health food stores are expanding their kosher selection of meats. For the moment, though, it may be necessary to order meat in bulk online or from local ranches. A good source for finding local, pasture-raised meats is eatwild.com. Glatt Kosher Grass-Fed is a company online that sells and ships kosher grass-fed beef, lamb, and poultry around the United States.

# Do You Need Supplements?

Even though the Paleolithic diet is full of nutrient-dense foods, we live in the modern world where soils are depleted of nutrients. Beyond that, after years of damaging our bodies by eating refined, non-Paleo foods, many folks are nutrient depleted and need supplementation. Should you take supplements while eating Paleo? It's a common question, and the answer is that sometimes supplements are a waste of money and sometimes they're not. Here are some of the supplements we recommend to people, depending on their situation.

## Multivitamins/Multiminerals

As we've said, our conventional soil is depleted compared with 100 years ago. On average, we're not getting as many nutrients from our food as our Paleolithic ancestors did, and eating organic will only help so much. We don't believe everyone needs a multivitamin/multimineral, but it sure wouldn't hurt to take one, as long as it's from a good source. A multi should not be used as a substitute for actual food, though: keep eating your fresh fruits and veggies!

We suggest you take a food-based multivitamin/multimineral, which means nutrients are extracted from foods so they're totally recognizable by your body (as opposed to some unrecognizable synthetic nutrients you'll find in many lower quality brands).

Studies have found that folic acid in fortified grains and most multivitamin supplements can actually cause cancer. It was thought that we could just convert the folic acid into the necessary folate in our bodies, but it turns out that's very difficult to do. What you want in your multivitamin, in order to avoid cancer and actually get the folate you need, are "natural folates," which come from food sources. Folic acid is part of the B vitamin complex, and it's important for brain and nerve function, as well as heart health and healthy pregnancy.

A few tips for getting the best products: look at the ingredient list for corn products (*dext-*), artificial colorings, or flavorings, and stay away from gimmicky, sugary supplements. All are warning signs of inferior products.

## Digestive Healing

Digestive complaints account for up to 40 percent of all doctor's visits. If you're like a lot of people, you may need a little help healing your gut. Of course, the best route to excellent gut health is eating Paleo. We've seen the diet completely eliminate reflux symptoms, bloating, diarrhea, and constipation, but a little extra attention is some-times in order.

> **DAMAGE CONTROL**
>
> If after a month of eating Paleo you're still having gas, heartburn, pains in your intestines, or other symptoms like headaches, acne, or fatigue, you might want to figure out if you have sensitivities to certain foods. Get tested for sensitivities by a nutritionist or naturopath or start experimenting with removing different foods from your diet and then adding them back in later. Remember that any food can have a negative effect on your immune system, from spinach to pork.

### Digestive Enzymes

Get a full spectrum of enzymes, including protease (for digesting protein), amylase (for carbs), and lipase (for fats), which can all come in one pill. Whatever brand you buy, make sure it doesn't have any corn (*dext-*) or other unnecessary ingredients in it. Take digestive enzymes as indicated on the bottle, at every meal and snack. They'll help you digest your food and allow you to start creating enough of them on your own again. You shouldn't need to be on digestive enzymes for more than a few months. In fact, it may only take a couple weeks for your own enzymes to start kicking in.

### Hydrochloric Acid

Hydrochloric acid (HCL) is what we use to start breaking down protein in our stomachs, and if you don't make enough of it you can experience gas, intestinal pain, heartburn, constipation, diarrhea, and fatigue after meals. It's an integral part of the digestive process and it is absolutely staggering that doctors constantly hand out purple pills to make it go away. It's usually not the overabundance of HCl that gives you heartburn; it's the lack of it and the mismanagement of it by your esophageal sphincter, which can be caused by eating certain non-Paleo foods over a lifetime.

You'll want to seek the council of a nutritionist or naturopath in order to take HCl correctly. When used properly, it can be incredibly beneficial to digestive problems. It can kick-start your body's ability to make enough of its own HCl. Keep in mind that like digestive enzymes, HCl is not a long-term protocol, and we believe the fewer pills the better.

### L-Glutamine

Glutamine has been shown in many studies to be one of the most effective gut healers available. It's an amino acid—you'd find it naturally in many protein foods—and it helps to maintain the tight junctions of the gut barrier. That means it helps to keep the walls of your small intestine from becoming leaky. Glutamine is a white powder with a slightly sweet taste that dissolves in water. Consult a nutritionist or a naturopath to find out if it's a good option for you.

## Bone Health

If you feel compelled to take a supplement for your bone health, just make sure it does not *only* contain calcium. It should also have some combination of vitamin K, vitamin D, magnesium, manganese, potassium, boron, zinc, and copper, all of which are necessary for bone health, too. Another very important aspect of bone health, besides getting enough protein, is using your muscles for weight-bearing exercise regularly. Exercise regularly to the point where you feel a burn in your muscles and get enough vitamin D from the sun or in supplement form.

## Individual Nutrients

You can take blood tests with your nutritionist, holistic MD, naturopath, or other alternative health practitioner that tell you which nutrients your specific body is low in. That could be anything from vitamin $B_6$ to magnesium to vitamin D.

Perhaps up to 90 percent of people are deficient in vitamin D. It's a buzz word in the nutrition and health world right now, and for good reason: vitamin D has a whole lot to do with bone health, heart health, immune function, and brain vitality, so if you're low in it, a lot can go wrong.

We mostly get vitamin D from being in the sun, but because we've been conditioned to apply sunscreen every day, people aren't producing enough vitamin D on their own. People certainly aren't eating much cod liver oil, mackerel, or sardines, either, which are some of the main food sources of vitamin D.

We're not saying you should go fry yourself in the sun all the time, but being out for an hour or so every day (without sunscreen) might just help increase your levels of vitamin D. The fact that many people stay inside every day, avoiding their vitamin D requirements from the sun may very well have something to do with the soaring rates of osteoporosis. And maybe that's why all of the calcium supplementation that's going on isn't doing much good: you need vitamin D to absorb calcium.

Get your levels of vitamin D tested to see if you're deficient (60 mg/dL or more is optimal). Ask your health-care professional how much to supplement if your levels are low. Experts are suggesting anywhere from 1,000 to 5,000 milligrams a day.

## Omega-3 Fatty Acids

Because most people have spent a lifetime loading up on inflammatory omega-6s at the expense of anti-inflammatory omega-3s, supplementing with omega-3s is a good way to play catch-up. The best sources of omega-3s are certain fish, fish eggs, fish organs (cod liver oil), and small crustaceans like krill. If you're going to supplement with omega-3s, we suggest you find a good source of krill oil, because it's a sustainable and clean source of the omega-3 fatty acids, eicosapentaenoic acid (EPA), and docosahexaenoic acid (DHA).

**NUTRITION FACT**

According to the USDA Nutrient Database, a 6-ounce serving of cooked wild Atlantic salmon contains 700 milligrams of EPA and 2,429 milligrams of DHA. Some of the highest quality omega-3 supplements provide 600 milligrams EPA and 400 milligrams DHA in a serving of two capsules. That means you'd have to take 3 capsules to get the equivalent of the EPA in the fish and 14 capsules to get as much DHA!

It also naturally contains a powerful antioxidant, astaxanthin, which not only helps protect you from oxidation, it preserves the oil itself, too. Fish oils encapsulated in capliques are superior to the normal gelatin capsules. They also protect the oil from oxidation. Get your fish or krill oil from a holistic health-care professional or a highly reputable source, either online or in your community. If you don't, you run the risk of consuming oxidized oils full of mercury and other pollutants. Store them in your refrigerator to maximize their life span. Don't leave them anywhere near your stove or out on the counter with the cap off!

Whatever supplements you end up taking, buy them either from a reputable health practitioner or a health food store. Many of the brands sold at conventional grocery stores and pharmacies are full of fillers and are low in the nutrients they claim to contain.

## The Least You Need to Know

- Raising a Paleo family can have its challenges, but time, patience, and open communication can create a smooth transition.

- Eating Paleo at least 85 percent of the time will keep you on track with your health goals, while giving you enough freedom to make the diet a sustainable lifestyle.

- While a strict vegetarian version of the Paleolithic diet might not get you to your optimal health goals, eating eggs and fish as your main protein sources can be very beneficial.

- Maintaining this diet while you're eating out or traveling is definitely possible if you follow some basic guidelines and plan ahead.

- You can keep kosher while eating Paleo when you find the right sources of meat.

- If you buy the right supplements, they can be helpful in certain situations.

# Paleo Nutrition for Athletes

## In This Chapter

- How our ancestors got exercise
- Using fat for fuel before a big race
- Making the diet work for endurance athletes
- Small modifications for the power athlete
- A 1-day sample menu for athletes

Compared with our hunter-gatherer counterparts, we are a lazy bunch of people. Most of us don't get adequate exercise every day because our lives are built around convenience and sitting. However, many of you get exercise by running, biking, weight lifting, or some other activity. And you need to know whether this diet is right for you. Don't you need tons of carbs to be a runner, and how do you get them eating Paleo?

Yes, you do need more carbs to be a high-intensity endurance athlete, but not as many as people might think. It's becoming well known that a lower carb, higher fat, and higher protein diet can help with weight loss, but it's not as widely accepted yet that the same kind of diet can benefit athletic performance of all kinds. The lack of refined sugars and grains and the lower omega-6 fatty acids all help to decrease inflammation, and that means fewer injuries and better performance overall. Paleo foods provide sustainable fuel to keep you from bonking, or having an energy crash, during your workout or race. Eating Paleo keeps your digestion working well so you don't have "emergencies" or side stitches during runs. And as you can see in Appendix E, you get plenty of nutrients to keep your whole body working optimally.

In this chapter, you find out how our activity levels differ from typical hunter-gatherers, and how you can make your own exercise program more evolutionarily appropriate. If you're an endurance athlete or a power athlete, you learn how to change the Paleo meal plan in this book to fit your needs. And finally, there's a sample menu for each type of athlete to help you visualize those changes.

# Hunter-Gatherer Activity Levels

We, like all other animals, evolved to only use the minimum amount of energy for the maximum gains. In other words, rest until you need to move around to find food was the M.O. of our forebears. After all, the calories necessary for getting up and moving weren't as plentiful as they are today. So it's our inborn tendency to do nothing until we have to. And today we don't ever *have* to do much, unless you're a construction worker or otherwise active at your job. All it takes is picking up your phone and ordering a pizza and voilà! You have yourself the equivalent of a day's worth (or more) of hunting and gathering, all without working up one single drop of sweat.

You could say that life was harder for hunter-gatherer groups, without phones (to order pizzas), dishwashers, laundry machines, cars, remote controls, baby strollers, Segues, elevators, and grocery stores. But they also didn't have 40-hour-a-week jobs keeping them from their family and friends, so it's a bit of a toss up as to which life is easier.

Primitive people spent their time walking, jogging, sometimes sprinting, climbing, carrying, jumping, crouching, digging, bending, building shelter, catching, throwing, swimming, crawling, and dancing, among other things. And don't forget having sex. Calories out (activity) roughly equaled calories in (food). On average, hunter-gatherers burned 800 to 1,200 calories every day in physical activity, which is three to five times that of modern sedentary people.

**PALEO COMPASS**

The American College of Sports Medicine and the Centers for Disease Control and Prevention laid out the following guidelines for physical activity to promote health: all healthy adults age 18 to 65 need to briskly walk for a minimum of 30 minutes, 5 days a week; jog for a minimum of 20 minutes, 3 days a week; or do some combination of the two. They should also do strength training at least twice a week. However, according to the 2003 National Health and Nutritional Examination Survey, in the United States only 3.5 percent of adults age 20 to 59 met those recommendations.

Let's compare our mostly sedentary lives to our ancestors. A typical hunter-gatherer exercise regimen did not include uselessly lifting weights to get ripped or running just for the sake of running. Activity was naturally born of daily chores, festivities, and socializing. The amount of activity varied by hunting and foraging practices, culture, weather, ages, and seasons. The following 13 basic elements of hunter-gatherer physical activity were laid out in *The Physician and Sports Medicine* by O'Keefe et al. in their 2010 paper, "Organic Fitness: Physical Activity Consistent with Our Hunter-Gatherer Heritage," which examined the activity levels of hunter-gatherers around the world.

- On average, they walked 3.75 to 10 miles a day. They walked to forage, hunt, gather water and wood, and sometimes to get to and from other villages. Lesson: move more.

- Difficult days were usually followed by an easier rest day, but they rarely took entire days off of all physical activity, because life depended on physical chores to provide for basic needs. Lesson: sometimes modern hardcore athletes are afraid to take a day off, but rest is necessary for good heart and joint health, as well as overall fitness.

- People walked and ran on softer natural surfaces, and almost never on solid flat rock or anything resembling concrete, as we do. They also didn't wear restrictive shoes like we do. Lesson: as expensive as your fancy running shoes are, the high heels and ill-fitting arches can actually do some serious damage to your body.

- Hunter-gatherers often needed to perform moderate to high-level intensity exercise punctuated by periods of rest. For instance, during a hunt they might walk, then see an animal and sprint, then walk again. Today, that's known as interval training (i.e., jog-sprint intervals or CrossFit). Lesson: you should do high-intensity interval sessions once or twice a week.

- They weren't specialists. In other words, they didn't train specifically to win a gold medal in squats. They were doing a variety of exercises, including strength, endurance, and stretching. Lesson: that sort of cross-training encourages overall fitness and reduction of injuries. It also keeps you interested in what you're doing and keeps you from burning out emotionally.

- They regularly did weight-bearing exercise like carrying heavy loads. Along with cardiovascular training, weight training is necessary for excellent health and fitness. Lesson: weight training, or just lifting heavy things in general, should be done at least two or three times a week for 20 to 30 minutes per session.

- Hunter-gatherers were usually lean, and that virtue alone reduced joint trauma and pain. Lesson: being lean and ripped isn't just good for attracting mates—it actually creates less pain in your body.

- They exercised outside almost all the time, where they were able to absorb the sun's rays to create crucial vitamin D. Lesson: it's healthier and more fun to work out outside than in a dank, dim gym.

- They often exercised in groups (hunting and foraging food, dancing, etc.). Doing difficult physical activities with other people can make exercise seem less taxing and it creates rewarding social bonds. Lesson: you might get more out of an outdoor soccer game than lifting weights solo in a stinky gym.

- Dogs and people have been evolving together for perhaps 135,000 years. Dogs have been domesticated for hunting, guarding, and transportation purposes, and that close relationship has not gone unnoticed by our genes. Lesson: it's been shown that exercising with dogs can help us stick with an exercise program, so if you have a dog, do him and yourself a favor and start walking and running together!

- They danced during rituals and other celebrations, sometimes several nights a week for hours on end. Lesson: dancing is fun *and* it's exercise. We should all do it more often!

- Sex is exercise, too, and hunter-gatherers obviously did that enough to successfully populate this earth. Lesson: sexual activity at least one or two times a week is associated with many health advantages.

- They gave themselves enough time for rest, relaxation, and sleep. Enough said. Most people today are over-worked, over-stressed, and sleep-deprived—all of which have tremendous health implications. So if you can, rest and relax more often!

The Paleo community generally regards these guidelines as hallmarks of healthy physical activity. In today's world, though, it's hard to burn a bunch of calories purely by doing chores, finding food, and socializing like our ancestors did. Most people spend the majority of every day sitting. Sitting at a desk, sitting in a car or train, sitting down to eat, and then sitting in front of a TV. The convenient life we've created for ourselves doesn't require much bending, climbing, or even lifting, so we usually end up picking a certain activity or two that we like in order to get exercise.

People find sports or workout regimes that fit their preferences and lifestyles. Maybe you play on a soccer league, or you rock climb, or maybe you go to the gym to lift weights. Chances are pretty good that if you exercise regularly, you run or bike. You may even be one of the serious endurance athletes out there. Eating Paleo can be effective for all kinds of athletes, whether you're doing power sports like weight lifting or endurance sports like long-distance running.

# Eating Paleo Fuels Activity

There's a common misconception among athletes that carbohydrates—particularly refined carbohydrates like sports drinks, pasta, and bread—are king. You supposedly need to load up on refined pasta before a big game or before a marathon. During the big game or race, you "need" to bring sufficient brightly colored sugar drinks in order to keep your energy up, and then you're told to eat a bunch of bread, cereal, or even pasta again after the event to make up for all that glycogen loss.

Conventional wisdom dictates high carb and low fat to athletes, but all that pasta and bread just create inflammation and extra body fat. Dietary fat is actually an excellent source of fuel for lower intensity endurance workouts, like most people's workouts are. It's true that endurance athletes need more carbohydrates, but perhaps not as many as you might think, and not at the expense of their health.

So what do you change about the Paleolithic diet if you're an avid athlete? The meal plan outlined in Chapter 18 fits sedentary to moderately active people better than serious endurance or power athletes. However, you can make small changes to the meal plan to get the fuel you need in order to perform your best and recover well.

# Tailoring the Diet for the Endurance Athlete

Endurance exercise is running, biking, swimming, and cross-country skiing, among others. When you're training for any of these activities 8 to 35 hours or more per week, you can consider yourself an endurance athlete. Anything less than that and you probably don't need to change the diet at all.

There is an argument in the Paleo world right now about whether endurance training is a healthy endeavor. Let's take a look at both sides of the argument so you can make an educated decision about whether it's right for you.

## The Case for Endurance Training

While some Paleo proponents caution against endurance training, or "chronic cardio," it seems it may be in our genes to be long-distance athletes. The proof is in our body mechanics. We have relatively little body hair and we sweat from glands all over our bodies to keep us cool. We can pant while running quickly, unlike many of our four-legged prey. And the bones and tendons of our feet and legs are supremely designed for running (barefoot or with simple shoes, that is). We also have this giant and efficient muscle in our derriere, the infamous gluteus maximus, which is mostly activated when running—not walking.

The San Bushmen of the Kalahari desert in Africa are known for persistence hunting, wherein they track an animal for many hours while running, walking, and sprinting, until the animal collapses from exhaustion. This type of hunting is thought to have been common long ago, because it's one of the most effective ways of killing an animal without a gun. That means we may have evolved doing long-distance endurance activities.

Paleo endurance running proponents use the Tarahumaran people of northern Mexico as ammunition for their case, too. The Tarahumaran people, who live semi-primitive lives, are known for regularly running up to 50 to 80 miles a day for persistence hunting, transportation, and communication between villages—all without shoes or with simple leather shoes. And all without one single drop of Gatorade. Amazing, isn't it? Seems like we're made to do this.

**PALEO COMPASS**

Men and women of the Tarahumara, young and old alike, have been known to run 435 miles in just over 2 days, during which time they burn a staggering 43,000 calories! To put that in perspective, the average marathon, which is 26.2 miles, costs runners about 2,600 calories.

## The Case Against Endurance Training

It's important to note that the Tarahumara tribe fuels up with fermented corn beer, which is something we could not have evolved eating because it's from a grain crop. The high carb content allows them to keep going and going. Their high-carb Neolithic fuel source is one of the arguments against intense endurance training while on a Paleolithic diet. It would take a lot of sweet potatoes to get you the carbs you need to run 50 to 80 miles a day, and you can only eat so many sweet potatoes ….

Also, persistence hunting, as it is traditionally done, is different from a professional marathon or a strict training regimen. Persistence hunters didn't run at constant Mach speeds for hours and hours when they were chasing an animal down: they were running at slow speeds with intermittent walking and sprinting. If you were a hungry hunter-gatherer chasing an antelope for 8 hours, you'd probably want to conserve energy, and slow speeds conserve energy. After all, you wouldn't even be looking forward to a high-carbohydrate meal to replenish your glycogen stores: more like straight up protein and fat from that antelope. Fat is an excellent source of fuel for low-intensity workouts, like persistence hunting (or a workout similar to it). We may have evolved running, but we probably weren't doing it like we do now, running at high speeds and high intensity many days of the week without proper rest.

But even if we were to say that high-intensity endurance training absolutely causes major health problems, a lot of die-hard endurance athletes would still do it most days of the week because they adore their sport. So whether or not endurance training is good or bad for you, we're going to tell you how to modify the diet to allow you to continue doing it—and to continue doing it really well.

## How to Modify the Diet

In a nutshell, to tailor the diet to an endurance athlete, you basically just add more carbohydrates and make sure to eat a high-protein meal before and after big workouts or races. By carbohydrates we mean Paleo carbs like sweet potatoes, potatoes (if you don't have an autoimmune disorder), tapioca, squash, fruit, and any of the other starchy veggies in Chapter 3. Let's delve into some details, though. We'll talk about what to eat before, during, and after a big workout or race.

## Eating Before Big Events

One of the biggest mistakes you can make is getting up after a night of sleep and doing a hard workout on an empty stomach. You're prolonging your overnight fast and burning some serious calories during your workout on top of it. You stimulate cortisol secretion, which inhibits proper recovery after your workout. Even if you *think* you do fine without breakfast before your morning run, just experiment with eating beforehand to find out how much better you could be performing—even if it's just a small snack.

**DAMAGE CONTROL**

Big workouts and races lasting over 90 minutes are times when even Paleo people use sports drinks or honey water (see the recipe later in this chapter). It would be difficult and damaging to go without this critical source of carbs. However, don't consume sugary drinks in the hour before your workout. Doing so may result in a blood sugar crash, leaving you weak and dizzy for your run. The only exception would be in the last 10 minutes before your workout begins. At that point, the extra sugar could benefit you because you'll be using it up as energy right away.

You want to eat a high-protein and high-carbohydrate meal before a big workout or race. What you're after in the protein are the amino acids, but especially the three branched-chain amino acids (BCAAs)—leucine, isoleucine, and valine. Consuming BCAAs before working out has been shown to increase the time it takes to reach exhaustion and the maximum energy you're able to output. The Paleo foods that are highest in the BCAAs are meat, fish, eggs, and nuts in that order. So basically, just eat any of the meals containing animal protein and you should be fine.

As far as the carbohydrates go, you need more of them for energy if you're working out an hour or more every day on average. For every hour of endurance work you do, an average person needs to take in about 50 to 100 grams of carbohydrates a day beyond what we recommend in this book. For reference, a large sweet potato contains around 40 grams, while a banana provides around 27 grams.

The more protein and fat you put into that preworkout meal, the slower the carbs will be released into your bloodstream, no matter what the source of carbs is. So if you're waiting two hours after you eat to run, consider having a pretty large meal, complete with Paleo carbs, meat, and a fat source. That's basically any of the meals we've laid out in the meal plan in Chapter 18, except you add more carbs.

If you're eating right before your workout, make the carb source simpler (less fiber and starch). Fruit will be easier to digest for most people than starchy potatoes or sweet potatoes, and the sugar will be more available right away for energy. As always, you'll need to experiment on yourself to see exactly how many carbs and from what food sources work best for you preworkout. It's different for everyone.

As far as the couple days leading up to a big event, it's not a big carb-loading bonanza like you may be used to. You'll want to eat normally, but put a serving of sweet potatoes, potatoes, or high-glycemic fruit like bananas into each meal and snack. That's enough to keep your glycogen stores topped off.

## Eating During Events or Big Workouts

You need to replenish calories and fluids during a cardio workout that lasts more than 90 minutes. It's often helpful to start the replenishing process before you reach the 90-minute mark to avoid bonking. For instance, you might want to start drinking something at or even before the 60-minute mark. Experiment to see what works best for you.

Eating solid food is often not an option for people when they're working out at a high intensity; digestion just doesn't work well at that point. People opt for sports drinks and sports gels chased by water, both of which are basically just simple sugars that are easily digested and quickly absorbed.

Even the strictest Paleo experts condone sports drinks and sports gels during long workouts over 90 minutes. Without a source of simple carbs, your body will start breaking down protein in the muscles for energy. You need those muscles—you can't go burning them for energy! Sports drinks also satisfy your need for water during long workouts, which is about 24 ounces per hour.

Consuming 10 to 20 grams of sugars every 15 minutes after the first 90 minutes of exercise can help keep energy levels up. You want to shoot for about 200 to 300 calories per hour. One typical sports drink every hour beyond the 90-minute mark will provide the calories *and* sugar you need. Sports gels and blocks are more calorie-dense than the drinks, so choose your products wisely. Also be sure to drink ample water with the gels or your digestion might suffer.

The other advantage to sports drinks, besides their digestibility and quick access to sugars, is their sodium content. When you're sweating for over an hour, you definitely want to replenish sodium and other electrolytes that are crucial for body functions.

Pick your sports drinks wisely and drink them only when you need to. While we are advocating them for endurance training, we're certainly not saying that just because you run 10 hours a week you should have a sports drink mustache all day every day. They're a compromise in this diet, so use them sparingly. Look for products with the lowest amount of preservatives, artificial flavorings, and artificial colorings. Or better yet, make your own out of honey or glucose, salt, and water. Here's a recipe:

# Honey Lemon Thirst Quencher

Recipe courtesy of The National Honey Board.

| Yield: | Prep time: | Serving size: | |
|---|---|---|---|
| 8 servings | 10 minutes | 1 cup | |
| **Each serving has:** | | | |
| 60 calories | 17 g carbohydrates | 0 g fat | 0 g protein |
| 119 mg sodium (electrolyte) | | 85 mg potassium (electrolyte) | |

½ cup honey

½ tsp. sea salt

¼ cup fresh lemon juice

7½ cups lukewarm water

1. Combine honey, sea salt, lemon juice, and lukewarm water and stir to dissolve honey.

2. Let cool or chill before serving.

**DAMAGE CONTROL**

Be sure to practice drinking and eating during long workouts before your big event. Figure out what kinds of sports drinks—homemade or store bought—work best for your digestion and energy levels. The last thing you want is a surprise upset stomach halfway through a race because you tried out a new drink or sports gel.

## Eating After an Event

In the first 30 to 60 minutes after exercising for over an hour, you'll want to replace some of the carbohydrates and protein you lost. It's actually a crucial time for carb and protein replenishment because your body is particularly receptive to those nutrients at that time. Studies have shown that eating immediately after exercising can help repair muscle damage and overall recovery. Because your digestion might be a little impaired right after a big workout, go for easily digestible foods like fruit, applesauce, a Tapioca Crêpe (recipe in Chapter 10), or even baby-food fruits because they're mashed up and easily digested. Baked yams and potatoes are a good option if you can stomach them. For protein, look to meat, fish, eggs, and nuts in that order.

This is the time when some athletes pressed for time will reach for egg white or whey protein powder. Protein powder is not the best option in our opinion, but it's easily used by your body if you can digest the dairy and it can be mixed with fruit and juice for a good balance of protein and simple carbohydrates. Some Paleo endurance athletes use homemade recovery drinks that include juice, protein powder, and honey. Consider these options only if you don't have time for a meal.

Be sure to hydrate after a long workout. If you weigh yourself before your workout, and then weigh yourself again afterward, you can get a feel for how much water you lost. For every pound of weight you lose, drink about 16 ounces of liquid. Then continue drinking your normal amount of water throughout the rest of the day, or even a little more, just to be sure to stay on top of your water needs.

After your immediate postworkout meal, just add a moderate amount of Paleo carbohydrates to one or two of your remaining meals and snacks for the day. Remember, you want to consume 50 to 100 grams of extra carbohydrates for every hour of endurance exercise, depending on your size and the intensity of your workout. Experiment with different amounts of carbs after long workouts. Watch how eating more or less affects your weight and performance goals. Everyone is different.

These suggestions apply to workouts or events that last from 90 minutes to 4 hours. When you move beyond that time frame, your water and calorie requirements change. For more information on the minutia of what you should be eating and drinking during ultra-marathons and IronMan distance races, or other very long-distance events, we suggest you read *The Paleo Diet for Athletes* by Loren Cordain and Joe Friel. It also provides a lot more detailed information on shorter races and workouts. Another good source of information is *The Paleo Diet Cookbook* by Nell Stephenson and Loren Cordain. Nell Stephenson is a very successful IronMan athlete and provides great practical advice on her website (nellstephenson.com) for endurance athletes. See Appendix B for details on both books.

# Tailoring the Diet for the Power Athlete

If you lift weights, box, wrestle, rock climb, or sprint regularly, you are a power athlete. Any athlete who values low body fat, strength, power, and stamina, as opposed to pure endurance, is a power athlete. Intense exercise of this kind three to five times a week, lasting an hour or less is what the Paleolithic diet supports naturally, without having to make compromises like sports drinks and gels.

If you're eating vegetables or fruits in most of your Paleo meals and snacks, then you're naturally providing your body with enough glucose to keep your glycogen stores full. What you don't get from dietary carbs can be manufactured in your body by protein and fat.

If you're doing power workouts more than three times a week for at least an hour each, you'll need to modify the diet a bit to keep your energy levels and performance at their peak.

Here are some guidelines for the power athlete:

- Make sure you're getting enough calories in general. A common mistake with athletes is eating too little, so if you start to feel fatigued regularly, increase your portion sizes.

- Eat at least 1 gram of protein per pound of lean body weight daily for optimal body composition and performance. If you weigh 135 pounds and you have 25 percent body fat, that means your lean body weight is about 101 pounds. You'd want to eat at least 101 grams of protein a day.

- Eat high-carbohydrate meals that include a generous serving of sweet potatoes, potatoes, or squash two or three times a week. This will help keep your body fat low and glycogen levels topped off.

- Eat Paleo fats liberally in your diet to ensure that your body has a good source of fuel beyond just carbohydrates. Remember, you don't want to use your muscles as fuel!

- Make sure you get a protein-rich meal or snack within 30 minutes after your workout to ensure muscle recovery. "Protein-rich" doesn't mean you eat a few nuts. You need all the different amino acids you can get, especially the branched-chain variety, so animal sources of protein are necessary.

Refer to Appendix B for more resources for the power athlete.

# Sample Meal Plans

Let's take a look at sample meal plans for an endurance athlete and a power athlete. We've noted the chapters in which the recipes are found.

## Endurance Athlete Sample Day

This sample meal plan is for a person doing a morning endurance workout lasting over an hour, or for a person who has an endurance event the next day.

### Preworkout Snack

- Small amount chicken or hard-boiled egg

- 1 to 3 cups melon or 1 cup berries

### Postworkout Breakfast (within 30 minutes of working out)

- Fried Eggs with Sweet Potato Hash (recipe in Chapter 9) *or* Sausage Stir-Fry Breakfast (recipe in Chapter 9)

- 1 cup berries and ½ melon

### Lunch

- Spaghetti (made with spaghetti squash and beef marinara)

### Snack

- Jerky

- Paleo Trail Mix (recipe in Chapter 11)

- Apple

### Dinner

- Almond Crusted Salmon (recipe in Chapter 13)

- Rosemary Green Beans (recipe in Chapter 12)

## Power Athlete Sample Day

This particular meal is not one of those high-carb days of the week. If it were, one of your meals would look like the endurance athlete's breakfast or lunch.

### Breakfast

- Shrimp and Avocado Omelet (recipe in Chapter 9) with extra avocado

- ½ cup berries

**Preworkout Snack**

- Chicken or hard-boiled egg; nuts

**Postworkout Meal**

- Pepper Steak (recipe in Chapter 14)

**Snack**

- Jerky

- Paleo Trail Mix (recipe in Chapter 11)

- Peach

**Dinner**

- Salmon with Coconut Cream Sauce (recipe in Chapter 13)

- Chard and Cashew Sauté (recipe in Chapter 12)

## The Least You Need to Know

- Hunter-gatherers generally did a lot more physical activity than modern people.
- Pasta and other refined carbs are no longer the only pregame meal; think protein and fat for fuel, too.
- Endurance athletes need to eat more carbohydrates and occasionally make compromises in their Paleolithic diet to maintain performance levels.
- Power athletes do well eating Paleo, but they should take special care to get the right amount of food at the right times.
- The sample menus give you a good idea of what your plate should look like as an endurance athlete or a power athlete.

# The Modern Kitchen Meets the Oldest Diet

## In This Chapter

- Revamping your kitchen
- Stocking up on staples
- Hassle-free mealtimes
- How much is this going to cost?

You're sold on this diet and you're determined to take back your health, take control of the food you put into your body, and get back in shape. There's just one small problem: your life and kitchen are set up for you to eat what you've always eaten and cooked (or not cooked) like you've always done in the past. In the process of taking back your health and waistline, you'll need to take back your kitchen as well. In this chapter, we teach you exactly how to do that, including what foods to get rid of, what to buy at the grocery store, and how to make preparing meals as easy as possible.

You may be wondering what all this is going to cost you. Will this new way of eating fit your financial situation? Most likely, it will. It doesn't have to be much different than what you spend on food now. If you decide to eat the most ideal, organic, and pasture-raised foods, it may cost more than what you're used to, but you can do this on a pretty tight budget if you need to. Now let's get to the kitchen!

## Out with the Old

Many restaurants don't offer many options for Paleo eaters, so you're probably going to find yourself spending a bit more time in your kitchen than you're used to. And because your kitchen is probably stocked with things Westerners—not hunter-gatherers—would eat, you're going to need to clean it out and restock it with Paleo-friendly foods.

The thought of throwing away your favorite cookies may have you asking, "Can't I just take this slowly? I don't need to totally revamp my kitchen just yet, do I?" Unfortunately, you probably should. Think about it. What's going to happen when you come home from work, a week into the diet when you're detoxing from your old way of eating, desperate for something to put in your mouth? In your low blood sugar delirium are you going to grab some raw nuts and a hard-boiled egg, or are you going to stuff your face with the chips you kept in your cupboard because you couldn't bear to throw them out?

> **PALEO COMPASS**
>
> Donate items such as canned goods and unopened packages to your local food pantry. If an item is opened or perishable, give it away or throw it away.

## Cleaning Out the Cupboards

It's time to make room in your kitchen for your new Paleo foods. The following list includes all dairy products, even though you may end up eating dairy later. We suggest you not eat dairy for the first month of eating Paleo in order to determine its effect on you. After the first month, return to eating dairy and see how you feel. For more information on the dairy debate, read Chapters 1 through 3. For now, here's what must go:

- Bagels, English muffins, and pastry
- Beans (black, garbanzo, pinto, etc.)
- Bread
- Breakfast cereal
- Cake/brownie baking mixes (even most gluten-free kinds)
- Candy bars and candies
- Canola oil
- Chips made with seed oils (potato, tortilla, pita, etc.)
- Cookies
- Corn products (tortillas, popcorn, corn chips, cereal, etc.)
- Crackers
- Most energy bars (containing oats, soy, refined sugar, etc.)

- Grain flours (white, all purpose, oat, wheat, rice, millet, etc.)
- Granola bars
- Oatmeal
- Pasta
- Peanut butter (to be replaced with almond butter)
- Peanut oil
- Refined olive oil
- Rice
- Safflower or sunflower oil
- Slim Jims or any other jerky product containing nitrites, preservatives, or unnecessary ingredients
- Soups containing grains, beans, corn, soy, vegetable oil, or dairy
- Soy sauce, tamari, and wheat-free tamari
- Sugar (sugar cane, brown, powdered, etc.)
- Sweetened condensed milk
- Vegetable oil
- Any food not listed here that is not directly derived from vegetables, fruits, meat, eggs, nuts, or acceptable Paleo seeds

## Cleaning Out the Fridge

Now move on to your refrigerator/freezer. As you open the door, think back on all the times you've stood in front of it, searching for that certain something that would satisfy your craving. And then look forward to the near future when it will be stocked with fulfilling, nourishing, and delicious options. Start bagging up the following:

- Butter
- Cheese
- Coffee creamers
- Frozen prepared meals

- Fruit juice; sports drinks (unless you're an endurance athlete); sweetened teas; and pretty much all beverages except filtered water, coconut water, and herbal teas

- Hummus

- Ice cream made with dairy

- Jams and jellies

- Margarine and other butter substitutes (Smart Balance, etc.)

- Meats containing nitrites

- Milk (including soy milk, oat milk, and rice milk)

- Soda (including diet soda with artificial sweeteners)

- Tofu/tempeh

- Yogurt

- Pretty much everything else in the freezer except frozen fruits and vegetables, meat, and seafood

> **PALEO COMPASS**
>
> If you live with others who aren't quite ready to take the Paleo leap, make designated spaces for your food so when you're looking for something to eat, you're not reaching past their tempting chocolate chip cookies to get to your beef jerky.

# Loading Up on Staples

Now that your kitchen is empty (and you're hungry from all that cleaning), what do you fill it back up with? And moreover, where do you get these things? You can find a list of staples you should always have on hand in Appendix C. It includes foods like fruits, veggies, eggs, meat, fish, nuts, and other less perishable items like almond flour, coconut oil, and various herbs and spices. The items on that list will help you make delicious, satisfying, and well-rounded Paleo meals and snacks. If you can find the items organic, we highly suggest purchasing those.

Be sure to check out Appendix B, where we share links to online sources for many of the staple items if you can't find them locally.

You can buy almost all of the staple ingredients at your local grocery store. The items you may have trouble finding there are the organic and pasture-raised products and the coconut products. For those, you may want to look into buying from local farms and ranches, at health food stores, or online.

While health food stores like Trader Joe's and Whole Foods are pretty common in major cities, you may not live close enough to one to shop there exclusively. Also, we recognize that health food stores are often more expensive, even for the exact same products. Here are some tips to keep in mind when shopping:

- Go for organic whenever possible. Organic foods contain more nutrients and no harmful pesticides or genetically modified organisms, which are both potentially harmful to your health. Organic farming practices are also better for the environment and the animals are generally treated better.

- Go seasonal for your produce. This will often be the fruit and vegetables on sale. It doesn't mean they're on clearance, but asparagus is cheapest when it's in season.

- Look for a "Natural Choices" section in conventional grocery stores. This may be called many different things depending on the store, but most major chains have at least one section where you can get less common and more natural food items. It can make shopping much quicker.

- For the most part, avoid the center aisles of a store. Traditionally, the healthiest foods—the fruit and vegetables, as well as the meat and fish counters—are on the edges of the store. The center aisles are often full of sugary drinks, candy, and highly processed foods and snacks.

- Try to find a local co-op or farmers' market for everything you can. Just because you don't have a Whole Foods nearby, you may still have healthier foods available.

# Making Mealtime Convenient

No matter what size your kitchen is, you need to make space for chopping, have tools and foods readily available, and make it easy to throw things away. You now have the food you need to make Paleo meals, so let's look at how to make mealtime easy and something you'll look forward to.

## Tools of the Trade

The following items will help make cooking easier, quicker, and less expensive in the long run:

- Extra freezer for storing goods bought in bulk
- Food processor
- Hand-held immersion blender
- Ice-cream maker (for coconut milk or nut milk ice cream)
- Meat smoker
- Vitamix blender (basically a blender on steroids)

## Easy Food Preparation

Before you actually go to make a meal, you'll probably need to prepare the ingredients in some way. When you're in a hurry, the last thing you want to do is chop up a bunch of vegetables and meat and *then* start cooking it. Fast can mean skimping on ingredients and going for less nutrient dense foods (i.e., skipping the vegetables), or fast can mean having everything already prepared in advance.

Take meat, for instance. You *could* cook one serving of chicken when you want a chicken meal. Or you could roast a pound and a half of chicken breast cutlets at one time. That way you can just take the already cooked chicken out of the fridge, throw it in a salad or sauté it with some vegetables, and have a quick dish. You can even eat cold meat straight out of the fridge with a little avocado spread on top—very quick and very satisfying.

What a lot of people don't realize is that cooking a bunch of meat at one time can be easy and fast. When you have small portions of meat, roasting takes very little time. For instance, roasting that pound and a half of chicken breast cutlets takes, at most, a whopping 14 minutes, 12 of which you can spend doing other things. Yep, 1 minute to put the chicken onto the pan, 12 minutes to roast it at 350°F, and 1 minute to take it off the pan and put it into a storage container. Okay, *and* another 30 seconds to clean up the pan. You can do this at any time of any day so you have a stockpile of chicken all week.

You can do the same, give or take a few minutes, with most steaks, turkey breast cutlets, pork chops, salmon, and many other meats.

> **PALEO COMPASS**
>
> Keep the foods you use the most at a height you can reach, or easily accessible in the fridge. Have a fruit and veggie basket on your counter if you have room, and keep it stocked. Keep your oils, spices, and other favorite flavor enhancers out on your counter, or easily accessible in a drawer or cupboard.

You can also save time by having a stash of already chopped vegetables in your refrigerator. Instead of having to chop up a serving of veggies every time you want them, you can chop them while you're waiting for some sauce to simmer, or while you talk to your kids about their day at school. Then just store them in the fridge. You'll be happy the next morning when you can prepare a giant veggie and chicken salad for the day's lunch in under 5 minutes.

In fact, whenever you're preparing or cooking any food, think about making more of it. For example, sweet potatoes take a long time to bake or boil. You may as well make two or three of them if you're going to take the time to make one. Hard-boiled eggs, salad mixes, trail mixes, muffins, jerky, and Tapioca Crêpe (recipe in Chapter 10) batter are all good candidates for making in bulk and storing for later. They all keep for at least a week.

## Easy Food Storage

Storing your leftovers is often a major part of the cleaning up process, and you can make that easier on yourself, too. To begin with, have an ample assortment of storage containers, preferably glass ones, on hand. Glass storage containers are easy to see through, so you know what you have in there. You won't waste time searching for food and you won't waste food (and money) by forgetting it's there. Glass also doesn't leach BPA, phthalates, or any other potentially harmful plastic chemicals.

Glass mason jars work well for storing nuts, seeds, coconut milk, and other leftovers. Small glass bowls with tight-fitting lids are great for transporting snacks the next day, and large glass bowls are perfect for storing big pot roasts or soups. You get the picture—just give yourself a lot of glass options and keep them organized so you don't have to spend a half hour trying to find matching lids.

# Fitting a Paleolithic Diet into Your Budget

You now know how to incorporate all of this into your kitchen, but what about your budget? Is this way of eating really feasible? If you want to eat the *ideal* Paleolithic diet that best mimics our ancestors, you would eat the following:

- Organic flours

- Organic fruits and vegetables

- Organic oils

- Organic, pasture-raised meats and eggs

- Raw, organic nuts

- Wild-caught or sustainably raised fish and seafood

However, those foods aren't cheap and there are plenty of places across the country where they just aren't available. In Appendix B we include websites where you can buy these products online, but with the shipping costs it often ends up being quite expensive. If you want to eat ideal Paleo, you may have to make some sacrifices in your budget elsewhere—that's up to you. However, you can make it work on a budget, too, by being thrifty, buying in bulk, or not eating all organic and pasture-raised foods.

So how much will this actually cost? Most people who eat this way spend $300 or less per person on groceries every month. Some people make it work on a budget of $125 per person per month. At most, if you ate the ideal foods without using any of the following money-saving techniques, you might spend up to $500 per average-size person per month.

To put this into perspective, the USDA suggests that an adult male spend anywhere from $166 to $330 per month on food in order to get enough to eat and be healthy (their version of healthy, that is). So it can be about the same as what you would be spending on a "healthy" Western diet.

Remember that you'll be eating out less now, so the money you'd normally spend at restaurants can be redirected to your grocery budget. Here are some more ideas for saving money on food:

- Grow it yourself. If you freeze, can, or jar a lot of what you grow, you can continue to save money throughout the year.

- Buy meat in bulk. Local ranches will sell you grass-fed beef by the quarter or half (or more) at a lower cost than regular retail. (See eatwild.com to find a ranch near you.) You could go in on something like this with a friend or relative and share the cost, which often comes out to under $3 per pound for all cuts. You can also ask around to see if anyone you know had an overly successful hunting season.

- Set up an account with a CSA (Community Supported Agriculture) at a local farm. When you have a CSA share, you receive a selection of local produce at regular intervals—every week or two—often at discounted rates. (See doortodoororganics.com or localharvest.com for more info.)

- Shop the bulk section in grocery stores for nuts, dried fruits, seeds, flours, and other items. It's often way cheaper than buying small, prepackaged bags. For instance, a pound of almond flour in bulk might cost as much as $4 less than if you bought a prepackaged, 1-pound bag of it.

- Raise your own chickens for eggs in your backyard. A lot of people are doing this now, and it's amazing how much you save on eggs if you do. Plus, your own hens will likely be much better fed and treated than conventional egg hens.

- If you don't have room or time for raising your own chickens, try to find a local source for eggs. They're often much cheaper when you buy directly from a farm or your neighbor.

## The Least You Need to Know

- Don't wait to clean out your kitchen; do it now while you're motivated so you don't have temptations later.
- Replenish your kitchen with staples like fresh produce, meat, fish, eggs, and nuts.
- Concentrate on the perimeter sections of grocery stores and read all ingredient labels carefully.
- Make your kitchen more efficient by creating space for food preparation and having an ample assortment of storage options.
- Cook and shop in bulk—it saves time later and takes less time than you'd think.
- Know that you can make Paleo work on almost any budget.

# Cooking Tips

## In This Chapter

- Making delicious, tender meat, poultry, and seafood
- Which oils and fats to use and when
- Paleo flours for baking and cooking
- The right ways to sweeten up the diet

Preparing and cooking meat and fish can be a daunting task to the uninitiated. When you go to a good restaurant and order a steak, a respectable, savory, perfectly heated cut of meat is served. But when you go home and try to re-enact that experience, it's easy to come up short. But with a little know-how, you can serve yourself up a restaurant-worthy piece of meat, too. In this chapter, we guide you through basic meat and fish cooking strategies.

Cooking meat may not be the only thing that's foreign to you about cooking foods on this diet. For instance, the flours, oils, and sweeteners in Paleo muffins are not typical. Instead of white flour, margarine, and white sugar, you'll use things like almond flour, palm oil, and coconut sap. We'll tell you where to get all of those foods and how to use them right.

## Preparing Meat, Poultry, and Seafood

The daunting idea of successfully cooking meat and fish is often what keeps people from eating them. We want to make sure we spare you the tragedy of missing out on such high-protein foods. Meat and fish are staples on this diet, but nobody loves stringy, tough meat. It's the tender, juicy stuff we all crave.

Here are a few general guidelines:

- Buy a meat thermometer. Thermometers take the guesswork out of perfectly cooking your meat. The desired internal temperatures of different meats are easily found on the internet or in any basic cookbook.

- Start cooking your meat, poultry, and fish when it's at room temperature. If you do, it ends up being tender and evenly cooked. Simply take the meat out of the refrigerator a half hour to an hour before you cook it.

- Make sure to pat the meat dry before you begin cooking unless you've marinated it. That will help to ensure even cooking.

Cooking breaks down the protein in meats, making it more digestible. Some argue that cooking meat makes it carcinogenic because it denatures the protein, but others contend that our brains wouldn't have evolved so extensively without predigested, cooked meat to help it develop. We say cook your meat, preferably to medium rare or below (despite the FDA's guidelines to always eat your meat well-done), but don't burn or char it. Burning meat produces *carcinogens*, and you don't want that.

**DEFINITION**

A **carcinogen** is any substance that is capable of causing cancer.

As a general rule, tender cuts (usually the more expensive ones) are cooked by dry-heat methods like grilling, sautéing, or roasting. Tougher cuts are best cooked by moist-heat methods like stewing or braising, where the long, moist cooking tenderizes the meat.

## Marinating and Tenderizing

Making meat tender is crucial. It's friendlier on the chewing muscles and it just tastes better. Marinating and tenderizing are two ways of achieving that before you start cooking the meat.

Marinate meat by letting it sit in a solution of liquid, oil, herbs, and spices. The liquid is often lemon juice, wine, vinegar, or some combination of those. The meat can sit in the marinade for minutes or hours, depending on the recipe. The acid in the marinade helps break down the meat, which makes for a juicy, tender end product. The key to a good marinade is the balance of spices, acids, and oil.

You can also brine meat to tenderize it, which is when you soak it in a salt solution. Physically pounding meat also makes it tender.

## Roasting

Roasting, or using the oven to cook meat, is best for naturally tender cuts like rack of lamb or pork loin. The meat is usually seasoned and placed in an already hot oven at around 400°F. The fat that seeps out of the meat can be poured back onto the meat throughout the cooking process, also known as basting. You can also baste with wine or stock to keep the meat moist. Basting is especially important for fish and poultry, which can dry out easily. Red meats like beef and lamb can be served pink in the middle, but never serve chicken or pork pink in the middle.

## Pan Roasting

This method is for tender cuts like rack of lamb, beef rib, or thick burgers that are too thick to cook completely in a pan. If you try to cook a thick cut of meat in a pan, it can end up being tough on the outside and rare in the middle. Brown the meat on both sides in a pan on medium to medium-high heat and put it in the oven to finish cooking. (Make sure you have an oven-safe pan.) The amount of time it's in the oven is dependent on the size of the cut and the type of meat. For instance, chicken and fish often take less time than some cuts of beef.

## Stir-Frying

Stir-frying involves quickly cooking tender cuts of meat at a relatively high temperature. Coconut, lard (pig fat), and tallow (rendered animal fat) work well in this case. Use a large frying pan or a wok, turn the heat up to medium or medium-high, and wait until a small piece of food sizzles when you toss it in the oil. If the oil or fat starts to smoke, it has reached its "smoke point" and is becoming oxidized and rancid. You've essentially burned the oil, and it should be discarded.

Use small, uniform chunks of meat and stir constantly. Normally, stir-fry recipes also include vegetables. You can cook the veggies at the same time as the meat, especially if it's tender meat that will cook quickly. Or you can cook the meat first, remove it while you cook the veggies, and then place it back in the pan when everything is just about done.

## Pan-Frying

Anytime you cook meat or fish in a pan with fat, or "fry" it, you need to use a fat or oil that will stand up to the heat. You can keep the heat at medium and use coconut oil, or go up to medium-high if you're using tallow or another animal fat. Which fat or oil you use depends on the flavor you want to impart to the meat. We discuss more about which oils to use at which heats later in the chapter.

Place tender cuts of meat in an oiled pan on medium or medium-high heat, turning now and then until it's done. You can use this method with tougher cuts of meat by slicing it into smaller portions, too.

> **PALEO COMPASS**
>
> You actually don't need to use extra fat or oil when you pan-fry meats. The oil keeps it from sticking and gives it more flavor, but it's not necessary.

## Pot Roasting

Pot roasting is done by cooking meat in moist heat for a long time, sometimes even an entire day. This method includes braising, which is cooking large cuts of meat with less liquid; or stewing, which is cooking smaller cuts with more liquid. You can use the oven and a high-sided pan or a Crock-Pot to make pot roasts. You can also use a large pot on a stovetop. Pot roasting works well with tougher cuts.

If you're not using a Crock-Pot, first sear the meat on all sides. Then sauté veggies and garlic in a pot and add wine or stock to it. Bring it to a simmer and add the meat to the pot and place the pot in the oven to cook low and slow.

The Crock-Pot is a more hands-off method that can save a lot of time. You can just place the meat and vegetables in the Crock-Pot and leave it to cook for the day. You'll want to sear the meat (pan-fry it just until the outside is browned) before putting it in the Crock-Pot to make it tender. You can also add broth or wine to the Crock-Pot to tenderize it.

## Grilling and Broiling

Everyone knows about grilling, but here's a tip: if you sear your steaks on the hot part of the grill first, then move them to an area of medium heat, you'll get steak that's crispy on the outside and juicy on the inside. Just make sure you don't burn it!

Like grilling, broiling is another quick, dry form of cooking meat, poultry, and fish. It uses the broiler, which is located at the top or the bottom of your oven. You'll generally want to move an oven rack up close to it and make sure the broiler is hot before you place the meat inside. Make sure you use a broiler pan to catch the drippings. The broiler is best for thinner cuts of meat, especially fish. But be careful not to burn the meat, as the broiler is very hot. Another way to use the broiler is to roast peppers under it if you don't have a gas stove.

# Acceptable Oils and Fats

We've mentioned a lot of new fats and oils so far that you may have never used before, like coconut oil, tallow, and even lard. You know what olive oil is, but have you ever used palm oil or macadamia oil? Coconut oil comes from the white flesh of the coconut, and it imparts a coconut-y, mildly sweet flavor to foods. It also has an uncanny ability to make eggs fluffy. Palm oil is similar in nature to coconut oil, but it comes from a different species of palm tree. Tallow is animal (usually beef) fat that's usually rendered and clarified by heating and straining it. Lard is pig fat that's clarified in the same manner.

All these oils and fats have different properties and are good for different uses. It can be hard to keep track of what oils and fats to use for what dishes. Before we dive into that, though, here's a primer on fats to help you understand why some oils are Paleo and why others are not.

## Oils and Fats 101

Fats and oils are made up of fatty acids, and fatty acids are named according to how many double bonds they have. The more double bonds, the more unstable the molecule. The more unstable the molecule, the more easily it is oxidized by air, light, and heat (i.e., cooking). And if it oxidizes easily, it's more likely to contribute to chronic inflammation and thus chronic diseases.

Saturated fatty acids (SFAs) have no double bonds because they are saturated by hydrogen atoms. Monounsaturated fatty acids (MUFAs) have one (*mono*) double bond. Polyunsaturated fatty acids (PUFAs) like the omega-6s and omega-3s have more than one double bond (*poly*). So in order of most to least heat stable, the fats line up in this order: saturated, monounsaturated, and polyunsaturated. In other words, you don't want to heat up an oil or fat that contains many PUFAs or it will oxidize and become rancid, and therefore contribute to your overall inflammation levels and risk of chronic disease. Saturated and monounsaturated fats are much more heat stable, so we stick with those for cooking.

Every oil or fat found in nature is actually a combination of the different fatty acids; there's not one that is completely saturated or unsaturated. In fact, the fats we think of as saturated, like lard, contain MUFAs and PUFAs, too. Lard is actually about 40 percent saturated, 45 percent monounsaturated, and 11 percent polyunsaturated.

**NUTRITION FACT**

Technically, cooking "oils" are liquid at room temperature while cooking "fats" are solid. You would think that coconut oil would be called coconut fat because it's a hard, white substance at room temperature. However, it comes from the warm tropics where it is a liquid at room temperature, so it's called an oil.

## When to Use Each Oil and Fat

We suggest you cook most often with coconut oil, tallow, lard, and olive oil because they have either low PUFA or high SFA or MUFA concentrations, or both. We know you were probably told your whole life that saturated fat and lard, in particular, are bad for you. It might be a little difficult to let that go, but we urge you to try it out and trust that 2.5 million years of evolution can't be wrong.

Good sources of tallow and lard can be hard to find at a grocery store, since most lard is hydrogenated. Next time you cook your organic, nitrate-free bacon, save the grease in a glass jar and use that to sauté veggies or fry your eggs up to medium-high heats. You can even buy good, pasture-raised, organic animal fat and render it yourself into tallow or lard. There are countless sources online to guide you through that process. Even if you just get organic fat from a butcher and cook it down, you'll be much better off than using conventional seed oils. For grass-fed sources of fat, go to eatwild.com or localharvest.com.

Another option for those people who choose to eat dairy is ghee. Ghee is clarified butter, so it contains only trace amounts of protein and lactose. It has a very high smoke point, meaning it requires a lot of heat for it to oxidize. You can use it for high-heat cooking, like frying or stir-frying. But you'll want to buy nonhomogenized ghee made from grass-fed cows, which you can easily find online or in health food stores.

The following table lists acceptable fats and oils on the Paleolithic diet, with guidelines for cooking temperatures for each. The temperature suggestions are based on the overall amount of PUFAs relative to the SFA and MUFA content. Notice that most of the oils in this table have a relatively low omega-6 to omega-3 ratio (O6:O3), which decreases our overall intake of omega-6s, and therefore our inflammation levels. Many of the oils and fats are also higher in SFA and MUFA than the conventional seed oils.

The oils that are marked "None" in the Cook Temp. column should not be heated. Their high PUFA and low saturated fat levels make them better suited for unheated usage, such as in a salad dressing. Be sure to store them all in a cool, dry place and discard any unused high PUFA oils after six months.

## Fatty Acid Composition and Cooking Temperatures of Paleo Oils and Fats

| Oil or Fat | SFA% | MUFA% | PUFA% | O6% | O3% | O6:O3 | Cook Temp. (Highest) |
|---|---|---|---|---|---|---|---|
| Avocado oil | 12 | 70 | 13 | 12 | 1 | 12:1 | None |
| Butter* | 51 | 21 | 3 | 2 | .5 | 4:1 | Med |
| Coconut oil | 92 | 6 | 2 | 2 | 0 | n/a | Med-high |
| Cod liver oil | 23 | 47 | 23 | 4 | 19 | .2:1 | None |
| Extra-virgin olive oil | 14 | 73 | 11 | 11 | 0 | n/a | Med |
| Flax oil | 9 | 20 | 66 | 13 | 53 | .2:1 | None |
| Ghee* | 65 | 32 | 2 | 2 | 0 | n/a | High |
| Hazelnut oil | 7 | 78 | 10 | 10 | 0 | n/a | Med |
| Lard | 40 | 45 | 11 | 10 | 0 | n/a | Med-high |
| Macadamia oil | 13 | 84 | 4 | 2 | 2 | 1:1 | Med |
| Palm oil (unrefined) | 50 | 39 | 9 | 9 | 1 | 9:1 | Med |
| Tallow | 50 | 42 | 4 | 4 | 0 | n/a | High |
| Walnut oil | 9 | 23 | 63 | 53 | 10 | 5.3:1 | None |

*Butter and ghee are dairy and should be avoided for at least a month, and only eaten after that if you can tolerate them. See Chapters 1 and 3 for more information on dairy.*

The following comparison table includes the most commonly used oils in the Western diet and their respective fatty acid concentrations. You won't be cooking with the typical Western oils, so we didn't include the cooking temperature in this table. It's interesting to note how the fatty acid compositions of these oils differ from the Paleo oils listed in the previous table. In general, their PUFA percentages are higher, their SFA and MUFA percentages are lower, and their omega-6 to omega-3 ratios (O6:O3) are higher. Also, because the oils in the following table are usually highly heated when they're processed, the fragile PUFAs are often already oxidized by the time they get to you.

### Non-Paleo Oils for Comparison

| Oil or Fat | SFA% | MUFA% | PUFA% | O6% | O3% | O6:O3 |
|---|---|---|---|---|---|---|
| Canola oil* | 7 | 63 | 28 | 19 | 9 | 2:1 |
| Corn oil | 13 | 28 | 55 | 54 | 1 | 54:1 |
| Cottonseed oil | 26 | 18 | 52 | 51.5 | .5 | 103:1 |
| Margarine** | 15 | 39 | 24 | 22 | 2 | 11:1 |
| Peanut oil | 17 | 46 | 32 | 32 | 0 | n/a |
| Safflower oil | 8 | 14 | 75 | 74.5 | .5 | 150:1 |
| Soybean oil | 15 | 23 | 57 | 50 | 7 | 7:1 |
| Sunflower oil | 10 | 20 | 66 | 65.5 | .5 | 131:1 |

*Canola's omega-3 to omega-3 ratio isn't bad, but there are other problems with it. See Chapter 3 for more information.*

**Margarine also contains 15 percent trans fats, which are associated with heart disease.*

# Paleo-Friendly Flours

Yes, you read that right—flours do exist on this diet! Flours open up the world of muffins, pancakes, breaded meats, cookies, and bread. You'll just make those things without the high glycemic flours everyone's used to using. Coconut flour and almond flour are the two main Paleo flours. The other one we'll add to the lot is tapioca flour, which is a major source of carbs for a large percentage of the world, including some hunter-gatherer groups. The following table breaks down how those flours compare to white, all-purpose flour.

**PALEO COMPASS**

You'll find that the Paleo flours are a bit more expensive than white flour, but because they're not a staple in the diet, you won't be using them all that often. They're well worth the price. They can all be found in health food stores and online, and they're starting to pop up in regular grocery stores, too.

### Flour Comparison Chart (per ¼ cup flour)

|  | White Flour | Coconut | Almond | Tapioca |
|---|---|---|---|---|
| Calories | 114 | 120 | 160 | 100 |
| Fat | 0.3 g | 4 g | 14 g | 0 g |
| Carbohydrates | 24 g | 16 g | 6 g | 26 g |
| Dietary fiber | 0.8 g | 10 g | 3 g | 0 g |
| Protein | 3 g | 4 g | 6 g | 0 g |

## Coconut Flour

Coconut flour, made from grinding up the dried meat of coconuts, is a gluten- and grain-free alternative to conventional white or wheat flour. It's actually defatted when it's made, so the fat content is pretty low, unlike coconut milk or coconut oil.

Coconut flour is very high in fiber—about 40 percent—and has a decent amount of protein. The fiber and protein in coconut flour help keep your blood sugar from spiking like it would with white flour.

Coconut flour lends baked goods a rich texture and a hint of natural sweetness. You can use it in all baked goods if you follow a few guidelines:

- Compared to other flours, coconut flour is dense and absorbs a lot of liquid, so you need to use less of it than other flours to get the same product.

- If you're going to use it with other flours, a general rule of thumb is to blend ¼ cup coconut flour with ¾ cup of the other flour.

- If you want to completely substitute coconut flour for another flour in a recipe, add four eggs for every ½ cup of flour. In the absence of gluten, the eggs act as the glue to hold the flour together. So if your recipe called for 1 cup of white flour, you would use eight eggs along with the 1 cup of coconut flour.

There are a lot of recipes out there now that call for just coconut flour. Here is a bread recipe that makes about six slices. You can see that with not even a cup of coconut flour, you end up with a substantial amount of bread. See Chapter 10 for other tasty recipes that use Paleo flours.

# Coconut Flour Bread

This is a slightly sweet, hearty bread to accompany any meal, or as a snack on its own.

| Yield: | Prep time: | Cook time: | Serving size: |
| --- | --- | --- | --- |
| 6 slices | 10 minutes | 40 minutes | 1 slice |
| **Each serving has:** | | | |
| 300 calories | 26 g fat | 8 g protein | 14 g carbohydrates |

¾ cup coconut flour

6 eggs, beaten

½ cup coconut oil

2 TB. raw honey

½ tsp. sea salt

1 tsp. baking powder

1. Preheat oven to 350°F.

2. Whisk coconut flour, eggs, coconut oil, honey, sea salt, and baking powder together in a large mixing bowl, or blend in a food processor until all lumps are gone.

3. Grease a bread pan with coconut oil and pour the batter in.

4. Bake for 40 minutes.

5. Insert metal knife into center of bread. If it comes out clean, bread is done.

6. Place on cooling rack and serve warm or cold.

## Almond Flour and Almond Meal

Almond flour, made from ground-up almonds, is another low-carbohydrate, gluten-free, grain-free alternative to white or wheat flour. Almond flour comes from blanched almonds (no skin) and almond meal comes from almonds with their skin intact. A lot of people can't tell the difference, and you can use them interchangeably in recipes.

> **DAMAGE CONTROL**
>
> You can make almond flour yourself by just blending up some almonds with or without blanching them first. But be careful: if you blend them for too long they'll turn into almond butter!

Almond flour has a similar consistency to white flour, but it's a bit denser and heavier. Like the nuts themselves, it can be used in both sweet and savory recipes because it has a distinct, nutty flavor. It produces baked goods that are moist and light. It doesn't require any sifting or kneading.

Almond flour has the same nutritional qualities as almonds, so it's high in healthy monounsaturated fat and vitamin E. It also contains calcium, iron, and dietary fiber.

You can basically use it as you would white flour, but a lot of recipes will call for more eggs than normal (again, to act as glue).

## Tapioca Flour (Tapioca Starch)

When you hear the word *tapioca*, it probably brings to mind pudding with little tapioca pearls in it. The little tapioca balls and the flour are made from the same plant, but the flour is finely ground. Tapioca comes from the starchy root of a woody shrub, and it is the third largest source of carbohydrates in the world. It's also known as cassava, yuca (not to be confused with yucca), and manioc. Unlike the other Paleo flours, it is *not* low in carbohydrates or high in fiber or protein. However, it is gluten free and doesn't contain antinutrients, so we like to use it. Sparingly.

> **PALEO COMPASS**
>
> Because it's so high in nonfibrous carbs, tapioca flour has an effect on blood sugar just like refined grains would. However, if you use it sparingly and in conjunction with fat and protein, its effect on your blood sugar will be buffered.

We really recommend this food to endurance athletes (see Chapter 6), who generally need more carbohydrates.

Tapioca flour has a very starchy consistency, like cornstarch, and it's basically flavorless. It gives foods that stretchy, chewy consistency lacking in many gluten-free foods. Normally it's used in a mixture of flours, but there are recipes calling just for tapioca flour (such as the Tapioca Crêpes in Chapter 10). You can substitute small amounts of other flours with tapioca. For instance, a good mixture for a muffin recipe that calls for 2 cups of flour might be 1 cup almond flour and ½ cup each of tapioca and coconut flour.

# Sweeteners

The following sweeteners are a very small part of the Paleolithic diet, but it's okay to indulge sometimes, especially if you're not trying to lose weight. "Sometimes" doesn't mean every day, though: we're talking once a week or less.

You can substitute the Paleo sweeteners for table sugar in all methods of sweet treat making. The only alteration will be that you'll use a little less of the liquid sweeteners than regular sugar (about two thirds the amount).

We suggest you stick with raw honey and coconut sap as your main sweeteners, and eat the others as rarely as possible. Raw honey and coconut sap have the smallest impact on your blood sugar and offer the most nutrients of all the sweeteners.

You can buy many of these products at regular grocery stores. Otherwise, they can be found at health food stores, local honey shops, or online.

## Raw Honey

Raw honey is one of the few sweeteners we know hunter-gatherers actually ate. "Raw" honey is not heated or processed in any way, so it contains all the vitamins, minerals, and beneficial enzymes it's meant to. It looks milkier than conventional honey (which is what you usually find in grocery stores). It has a glycemic index of about 30, compared to refined honey at 75. Raw honey is the preferred Paleo sweetener.

**NUTRITION FACT**

Raw honey contains particles of bee pollen, honeycomb, propolis, and bee wing fragments, which may sound funny, but all of those things contribute to its impressive nutrient profile. It's very high in antioxidants, and some of its properties actually help digest carbohydrates. Refined honey has all of that goodness filtered out.

## Coconut Sap

Coconut sap, which also comes in its granulated form as coconut "sugar," is a low-glycemic (about 35, compared to table sugar at 70) sweetener derived from the nectar of the flower clusters of coconut trees. It's an environmentally sustainable source of food and it contains B vitamins, vitamin C, and inulin, a prebiotic fiber. Prebiotic means that it feeds the good bacteria in your gut. Coconut sap also comes in its dried, or granulated, form—coconut sugar.

## Stevia

Stevia is a plant that actually benefits blood sugar control by increasing insulin's effectiveness. But don't be fooled by some products that tout stevia as the sweetener: always read the ingredient labels, as they may have just added stevia to an arsenal of other toxic sweeteners. Also, stevia is usually sold in packets with corn sugar (maltodextrin or dextrin) added to them, in which case you're actually consuming sugar, not just stevia. We say go ahead and eat stevia, but only if it's truly just stevia, and watch for non-Paleo additives in the ingredient list of the products it's in.

## The Least You Need to Know

- It just takes a little know-how to cook a juicy, tender piece of meat.
- All fats and oils are made up of a combination of fatty acids, and those containing a lot of polyunsaturated fats should not be used in cooking.
- The acceptable flours to use in baking and breading are almond flour, coconut flour, and tapioca flour.
- Sweeteners should be used sparingly, but opt for raw honey and coconut sap when you do indulge your sweet tooth.

# Paleo-Perfect Recipes

If you're driving around lost in a storm far away from home, all you want is a GPS system with a soothing British voice to tell you which way to go, right? In the midst of removing some of your favorite foods and replacing them with some ingredients you've never even heard of before, you may feel like you're in that car lost without a GPS. We can't offer you the soothing British accent, but allow us to provide you with at least a road map: recipes.

In this part, we introduce you to over 100 recipes. With them, you'll never be at a loss for a delicious breakfast, snack, appetizer or side, dinner, or dessert. These satisfying dishes are made with simple ingredients and are often quick to prepare. They use the most recognizable Paleo ingredients to help make your transition to Paleo a smooth one.

# Savory Breakfasts

## In This Chapter

- Hearty omelets, frittatas, and scrambles
- New takes on old favorites
- Veggies are for breakfast, too
- Bacon lovers, rejoice!

Breakfast literally means to "break" your overnight "fast." It seems logical that you'd want a big, satisfying meal after not eating for an entire night. However, it's becoming more and more common to have a high-carb, refined-grain breakfast in a lot of cultures, like cereal or bagels in the United States, juice and bread with sweetened milk in Chile, or flatbread and jam in Iran.

On the other hand, hunter-gatherer societies eat hearty, unprocessed foods for breakfast—the same foods they eat for all their other meals. For instance, the Malaysian Batek people might have fruit, leafy vegetables, and monkey meat, and the Nukak people in the Republic of Colombia might have monkey meat, bird eggs, toucans, or catfish to break their fast.

We're not suggesting you go to the Amazon and catch a toucan for breakfast every morning! But we do encourage you to start thinking outside the (cereal) box and consider heartier, more blood sugar–balancing foods for breakfast. Meat, eggs, and vegetables are all fantastic breakfast foods. When you first start eating Paleo, it may be strange to think of savory foods you'd normally eat for dinner as breakfast. But as time goes on, it will become more normal and you'll start to enjoy the sustained energy those foods provide.

The savory breakfasts in this chapter will make you want to throw away those cereal boxes forever!

# Baked Eggs in Bacon Rings

The sturdy bacon holds all the vegetables in place, and allows you to taste the entire gamut of flavors in each bite. The mushrooms and onions pack a punch when cooked in the remaining bacon fat.

| Yield: | Prep time: | Cook time: | Serving size: |
| --- | --- | --- | --- |
| 4 bacon cups | 15 minutes | 20 minutes | 2 bacon cups |
| **Each serving has:** | | | |
| 555 calories | 13 g carbohydrates | 47 g fat | 22 g protein |

6 strips bacon

⅓ cup onions, chopped

4 white button mushrooms, chopped

1 medium tomato, cut into 4 thick slices

4 medium eggs

½ tsp. freshly ground black pepper

1. Preheat oven to 325°F.

2. Cook bacon in a skillet over medium heat until it begins to shrivel (about 3 minutes). Remove bacon from the pan and set aside.

3. Discard all but a shallow film of bacon fat in the bottom of the skillet.

4. Brush 4 cups in a muffin tin or 4 small ramekins with bacon fat from the pan.

5. Add chopped onions and mushrooms to the hot pan with remaining bacon drippings in the skillet and cook over medium heat until softened.

6. Place 1 tomato slice in the bottom of each cup. Circle the inside of each cup with 1½ strips of cooked bacon.

7. Break 1 egg into each muffin cup and season with pepper.

8. Add sautéed mushrooms and onions over egg.

9. Fill any unused tins with water to protect from burning.

10. Bake in oven for 20 minutes.

11. To serve, loosen the edges of eggs with a spatula and transfer eggs to plates.

**PALEO COMPASS**

It takes a little practice to get the bacon cooked just right so that you can properly line the cups with the bacon. It's better to leave it a bit undercooked than too crispy, or it won't be flexible enough to fit in the cup. Also, buying higher-quality, lower-fat content bacon will keep the bacon strips from shrinking too much, and they'll be thicker and sturdier while eating.

# Chorizo Scrambled Eggs

The spiciness of chorizo blends well with the eggs and onions, while the coconut oil offers just a hint of mild sweetness.

| Yield: | Prep time: | Cook time: | Serving size: |
|---|---|---|---|
| 3 cups | 5 minutes | 10 minutes | 1½ cups |
| **Each serving has:** | | | |
| 462 calories | 13 g carbohydrates | 33 g fat | 24 g protein |

½ medium yellow onion, diced

4 oz. hard chorizo, sliced

1 TB. coconut oil

4 medium eggs

¼ tsp. sea salt

¼ tsp. freshly ground black pepper

1 tsp. hot pepper sauce

1. Over medium-high heat, sauté yellow onion and chorizo in coconut oil until chorizo gets crispy around the edges and onion turns slightly translucent.

2. Beat eggs in a small bowl and add sea salt and black pepper.

3. Pour eggs into the pan with chorizo and onions.

4. Scramble eggs softly until cooked.

5. Top with hot sauce and serve hot.

**PALEO COMPASS**

Chorizo is a broad term for a spicy sausage, but is traditionally made in the Spanish or Mexican style. Spanish chorizo is usually a harder sausage that can be sliced and served in chunks. Mexican chorizo is more often ground and falls apart when outside the casing. This recipe works well with either, so experiment and find which you prefer.

# Eggs with Avocado and Salsa

This simple recipe doesn't lack flavor. The heat of the salsa is balanced with creamy avocado, and almonds add the perfect crunch.

| Yield: | Prep time: | Cook time: | Serving size: |
|---|---|---|---|
| 2 cups | 3 minutes | 5 minutes | 1 cup |
| **Each serving has:** | | | |
| 415 calories | 13 g carbohydrates | 32 g fat | 21 g protein |

| | |
|---|---|
| 4 medium eggs | ½ medium avocado, sliced |
| ½ cup sliced or slivered almonds | 4 TB. organic salsa |

1. Heat a nonstick skillet over medium-high heat.

2. Beat eggs in a small bowl and pour into the skillet.

3. Cook for 1 minute and turn heat to medium-low.

4. Finish cooking (about 2 to 4 minutes longer).

5. Dish it up with almonds, avocado, and salsa.

**Variation:** Spice up this recipe further with sliced jalapeños, black olives, cherry tomatoes, garlic, or fresh cilantro. Any of the usual taco toppings will make this dish stand out.

# Fried Eggs with Sweet Potato Hash

While not a typical, high-sugar breakfast, the sweet potatoes in this recipe bring out a subtle flavor that pairs well with the peppery fried eggs and salty sausage.

| Yield: | Prep time: | Cook time: | Serving size: |
|---|---|---|---|
| 5 cups | 10 minutes | 20 minutes | 2½ cups |

| Each serving has: | | | |
|---|---|---|---|
| 399 calories | 26 g carbohydrates | 25 g fat | 18 g protein |

2 TB. coconut oil

1 medium sweet potato or yam, diced into ½-in. cubes

½ medium yellow onion, diced

2 sausages, sliced

1 medium bell pepper, diced

1 TB. water

4 medium eggs

Freshly ground black pepper

1. In a large skillet, heat 1 tablespoon coconut oil over medium heat.

2. Add sweet potato and yellow onion, and sauté for 5 minutes.

3. Add sausages and continue to cook until sausages are browned and sweet potatoes are slightly softened.

4. Add bell pepper and water.

5. Cover and cook for 15 minutes or until sweet potatoes are completely soft, stirring frequently.

6. While dish is cooking, fry eggs in remaining 1 tablespoon coconut oil.

7. Season eggs with black pepper and serve hot over sweet potato hash.

# Ham and Applesauce with Almonds

The sweet and salty flavors from the applesauce and ham make a complex flavor profile that is complemented well by the almonds.

| Yield: | Prep time: | Serving size: | |
|---|---|---|---|
| 2 ham steaks and 2 cups applesauce | 5 minutes | 1 piece ham and 1 cup applesauce | |
| **Each serving has:** | | | |
| 600 calories | 480 g carbohydrates | 31 g fat | 42 g protein |

12 oz. ham

2 cups unsweetened applesauce

1 cup almonds

1. Slice ham and warm in a skillet on the stove (or eat cold).

2. Serve with applesauce and almonds.

# Myra's Chopped Mushrooms, Eggs, and Onions

This recipe is for bacon lovers. Eat it warm, or let the flavors meld as it cools in the refrigerator.

| Yield: | Prep time: | Cook time: | Serving size: |
|---|---|---|---|
| 8 cups | 10 minutes | 20 minutes | 2 cups |

| Each serving has: | | | |
|---|---|---|---|
| 522 calories | 6 g carbohydrates | 49 g fat | 19 g protein |

8 slices bacon

1 medium onion, finely diced

12 medium white mushrooms, finely chopped

8 hard-boiled eggs, peeled and finely chopped

Freshly ground black pepper

1. Cook bacon fully and remove from pan. Reserve a light coating of bacon fat in the pan. When cool, crumble bacon into pieces and set aside.

2. Over medium-high heat, sauté onion in remaining bacon drippings until translucent and golden brown.

3. Add white mushrooms and sauté another 5 to 6 minutes, stirring frequently, until softened.

4. Mix onion, eggs, and bacon together, and season with pepper. Serve warm or cold.

**PALEO COMPASS**

While people have traditionally wanted to cook their vegetables in bacon fat, most people have been told over the past few years that you shouldn't. However, as we've found, when eating grass-fed meat accompanied with a Paleo diet, you can fully indulge in appreciation of animal fat. No need to wipe the pan clean before cooking the veggies.

# Omelet Muffins

The salty ham is a lean protein that plays nicely with the savory muffins, asparagus, and creamy eggs.

| Yield: | Prep time: | Cook time: | Serving size: |
|---|---|---|---|
| 16 muffins | 10 minutes | 20 minutes | 4 muffins |
| **Each serving has:** | | | |
| 370 calories | 4 g carbohydrates | 29 g fat | 24 g protein |

16 medium eggs

16 oz. ham, cut into small pieces

4 cups diced, raw asparagus (or other vegetables such as broccoli, mushrooms, or bell peppers)

¼ tsp. salt

⅛ tsp. freshly ground black pepper

1. Preheat oven to 350°F.

2. Grease 8 muffin cups with coconut oil or line with paper baking cups. Fill any remaining muffin cups with 1 inch of water so they do not scorch while baking.

3. Beat eggs in a medium bowl and add ham, asparagus, salt, and pepper.

4. Pour mixture into the muffin cups.

5. Bake for 18 to 20 minutes.

6. Cool slightly, then remove from pan. Serve warm or cold.

**NUTRITION FACT**

These are a fantastic dish that can be made any time and heated whenever a quick snack is needed. They're very low in carbohydrates, so a piece of fresh fruit is an excellent accompaniment.

# Roasted Pepper and Sausage Omelet

The roasted poblanos in this dish provide plenty of rich peppery flavor without being too hot. The mild flavor is a perfect complement to the sausage, which can also be somewhat spicy.

| Yield: | Prep time: | Cook time: | Serving size: |
|---|---|---|---|
| 2 omelets | 10 minutes | 20 minutes | 1 omelet |

| Each serving has: | | | |
|---|---|---|---|
| 308 calories | 6 g carbohydrates | 23 g fat | 22 g protein |

| | |
|---|---|
| 1 poblano pepper | 2 tsp. coconut oil |
| 4 medium eggs | 4 sausage links, cooked and sliced |
| 1 tsp. freshly ground black pepper | 2 TB. fresh parsley, chopped |

1. Place poblano pepper in a heavy-bottomed pan over high heat. Turn pepper as skin begins to blacken and blister on each side.

2. When blistered on all sides, remove from the pan and put in a plastic bag with a few drops of water; seal the bag immediately with plenty of air trapped inside.

3. Wait 5 minutes. Remove pepper from the bag, cut out seeds, remove skin, and dice.

4. Beat eggs in a small bowl and add black pepper.

5. Heat a medium, nonstick skillet over medium heat. Add 1 teaspoon coconut oil when hot.

6. Add half of egg mixture to the hot pan. As egg starts to set, add 2 sausages, 1 tablespoon parsley, and half of pepper mixture to one half of the pan.

7. When fully set, fold half of egg over filling, and cook 1 minute more.

8. Repeat the process with remaining 1 teaspoon coconut oil, remaining half egg mixture, remaining 2 sausages, remaining 1 tablespoon parsley, and remaining pepper mixture to make the second omelet.

9. Transfer to dish and serve.

**Variation:** Depending on your preference, you can substitute the poblano pepper with something more mild, such as a green bell pepper or an Anaheim pepper. Or use a few jalapeños for more heat.

# Sausage Stir-Fry Breakfast

The spicy sausage and sweet coconut oil contribute the most prominent flavors to this easy breakfast. The greens also help give it a fresh balance to keep it from being too heavy.

| Yield: | Prep time: | Cook time: | Serving size: |
| --- | --- | --- | --- |
| 2 cups | 3 minutes | 10 minutes | 1 cup |

| Each serving has: | | | |
| --- | --- | --- | --- |
| 237 calories | 7 g carbohydrates | 15 g fat | 21 g protein |

1 tsp. coconut oil

½ medium yellow onion, diced

8 oz. sausage, sliced

4 cups spinach

1. Heat a skillet over medium heat, and add coconut oil when hot.

2. Add yellow onion and sauté until slightly translucent.

3. Add sausage and cook until browned, tossing frequently.

4. Add spinach, reduce heat to medium-low, and cover.

5. Serve when spinach is wilted and soft (about 5 minutes).

**PALEO COMPASS**

This recipe assumes the sausage is raw. If the sausage is precooked, add it once the onions are a few minutes away from being done.

# Savory Zucchini Fritters

Eat these fritters plain, or add a spoonful of raw honey for a sweet and salty flavor combination.

| Yield: | Prep time: | Cook time: | Serving size: |
|---|---|---|---|
| 4 (6-in.) fritters | 10 minutes | 10 minutes | 2 fritters |

| Each serving has: | | | |
|---|---|---|---|
| 228 calories | 10 g carbohydrates | 19 g fat | 15 g protein |

| | |
|---|---|
| 3 medium eggs | ½ tsp. sea salt |
| 1 TB. coconut flour | ¼ tsp. freshly ground black pepper |
| 2 medium zucchini, shredded | 1 TB. coconut oil |

1. In a large bowl, beat eggs together.

2. Sift coconut flour into eggs and beat together. Note: coconut flour often has clumps, which is why it is important to sift it.

3. Mix in zucchini, sea salt, and pepper.

4. Set a large skillet over medium-low heat. Add coconut oil to coat the bottom of the pan once it is hot.

5. Spoon the mixture into the pan in 6-inch fritters.

6. Cook until golden brown. Flip fritter and continue to cook until outside is golden brown and inside is fully cooked (about 5 minutes per side).

7. Serve warm or at room temperature.

**PALEO COMPASS**

These quick fritters are so delicious, you'll wish there were more! Make a double batch and save the leftovers for a tasty snack.

# Scrambled Eggs with Bacon and Vegetables

This hearty scramble is filled with the vibrant flavors of the green vegetables, while combining the savory and salty flavors of bacon.

| Yield: | Prep time: | Cook time: | Serving size: |
| --- | --- | --- | --- |
| 4 cups | 5 minutes | 20 minutes | 2 cups |
| **Each serving has:** | | | |
| 315 calories | 7 g carbohydrates | 21 g fat | 25 g protein |

| | |
| --- | --- |
| 4 bacon slices | 1 medium tomato, diced |
| 1 medium zucchini, diced | 4 eggs |
| 1 clove garlic, minced | 1 cup fresh spinach |

1. Cook bacon, remove from pan, and let drain on paper towels. Reserve 1 tablespoon of bacon drippings in the pan.

2. Crumble bacon and set aside.

3. Over medium-high heat, add zucchini, garlic, and tomato to the pan with bacon drippings. Sauté until just before tender.

4. Beat eggs in a small bowl and set aside.

5. When vegetables are almost done, add beaten eggs and crumbled bacon to the pan, along with fresh spinach.

6. Turn heat to medium-low and cook until eggs are fluffy and firm. Serve hot.

# Shrimp and Avocado Omelet

The texture of the plump shrimp and creamy avocado make this breakfast stand out. Cilantro and a hint of coconut oil give it a fresh boost in flavor.

| Yield: | Prep time: | Cook time: | Serving size: |
|---|---|---|---|
| 2 omelets | 10 minutes | 15 minutes | 1 omelet |
| **Each serving has:** | | | |
| 317 calories | 7 g carbohydrates | 23 g fat | 21 g protein |

| | |
|---|---|
| 4 oz. shrimp, peeled | ¼ tsp. sea salt |
| 1 medium tomato, diced | ¼ tsp. freshly ground black pepper |
| ½ avocado, diced | 1 TB. coconut oil |
| 1 TB. fresh cilantro, chopped | 4 medium eggs, beaten |

1. Cook shrimp over medium heat until pink. Chop and set aside.

2. Toss tomato, avocado, and cilantro together in a small bowl. Season with sea salt and pepper. Set aside.

3. Beat eggs in a separate small bowl.

4. Heat a nonstick skillet over medium-high heat. Add coconut oil when hot.

5. Pour 2 eggs into the hot skillet, tilting the pan gently to cover the bottom with egg. Tilt pan and lift edges of omelet to allow uncooked egg to spread to the hot part of the pan.

6. When eggs are almost fully firm, add 2 ounces shrimp pieces into one half of the pan.

7. Fold omelet in half and cook for a minute more.

8. Top with half of tomato-avocado mixture.

9. Repeat the process with the remaining 2 eggs, remaining 2 ounces shrimp pieces, and remaining half tomato-avocado mixture to make the second omelet.

10. Transfer to plate and serve hot.

**PALEO COMPASS**

You can often save time and hassle by getting precooked and frozen shrimp from many stores. Use these in a pinch to facilitate a quick and healthy breakfast.

# Summer Vegetable Frittata

With peppers, zucchinis, and a variety of fresh herbs, this dish is bursting with green flavors reminiscent of summer.

| Yield: | Prep time: | Cook time: | Serving size: |
|---|---|---|---|
| 1 frittata | 10 minutes | 25 minutes | ½ frittata |
| **Each serving has:** | | | |
| 456 calories | 16 g carbohydrates | 32 g fat | 10 g protein |

1½ TB. coconut oil

1 medium zucchini, diced

½ medium red bell pepper, diced

½ medium red onion, diced

1 TB. fresh thyme

½ tsp. sea salt

¼ tsp. freshly ground black pepper

2 garlic cloves, minced

1 medium tomato, seeded and chopped

9 large eggs

1. Heat coconut oil in a 10-inch, oven-proof skillet over medium heat. When hot, add zucchini, red bell pepper, red onion, thyme, ¼ teaspoon sea salt, ⅛ teaspoon black pepper, and garlic.

2. Cover and cook until vegetables are tender (about 5 to 7 minutes), stirring occasionally.

3. Stir in tomato. Cook, uncovered, for 5 minutes more or until liquid evaporates.

4. Combine eggs and remaining ¼ teaspoon sea salt and remaining ⅛ teaspoon black pepper and whisk until frothy.

5. Pour eggs over vegetable mixture and stir gently. Cover, reduce heat, and cook 15 minutes.

6. Preheat the broiler to low. Finish frittata with 3 minutes under the broiler, or until fully set.

7. Invert onto a plate, slice, and serve warm or cold.

**Variation:** Like an omelet, a frittata is open to interpretation. Feel free to add sausage, ham, or bacon for a bit more protein. However, be careful not to add too many extra juicy vegetables, as the egg may not set properly with the added liquid.

# Veggies and Eggies

Avocados, bacon, and kale provide a nice breadth of flavors, but the garlic is what really makes this dish a flavorful treat.

| Yield: | Prep time: | Cook time: | Serving size: |
| --- | --- | --- | --- |
| 4 cups | 5 minutes | 25 minutes | 2 cups |
| **Each serving has:** | | | |
| 584 calories | 81 g carbohydrates | 48 g fat | 19 g protein |

4 strips bacon

¼ yellow onion, diced

1 clove garlic, minced

4 leaves kale

4 medium eggs

1 avocado, sliced

1. Cook bacon. Remove from the pan and put on a paper towel to absorb extra oil. When cool, crumble bacon and set aside.

2. Drain the pan of all but a coating of bacon grease.

3. Sauté yellow onion in bacon grease until slightly translucent. Add garlic and kale to the pan, and continue to cook until tender. Use a slotted spoon to remove mixture to 2 plates.

4. With the pan still hot, cook eggs over easy in the leftover juices of the sauté.

5. When eggs are cooked, layer them on top of vegetables.

6. Top with avocado and crumbled bacon and serve.

**Variation:** The kale is easily replaced by chard or spinach, depending on what you have on hand, or is in season. However, don't leave it out altogether and neglect the benefits of a nice dark green-leaf veggie to add flavor and vitamins.

# Western Omelet

Classic flavors make this breakfast easy to enjoy and simple to make.

| Yield: | Prep time: | Cook time: | Serving size: |
| --- | --- | --- | --- |
| 2 omelets | 5 minutes | 15 minutes | 1 omelet |
| **Each serving has:** | | | |
| 284 calories | 9 g carbohydrates | 19g fat | 23 g protein |

½ medium yellow onion, diced

1 green bell pepper, diced

1 medium tomato, diced

1 cup spinach

4 medium eggs

1 tsp. coconut oil

¼ lb. ham, cooked and diced

¼ tsp. sea salt

¼ tsp. freshly ground black pepper

1. Wash and chop yellow onion, bell pepper, tomato, and spinach. Set aside.

2. Crack eggs into a small bowl and beat well. Set aside.

3. Heat a nonstick skillet over medium heat. When hot, add coconut oil to the pan.

4. Pour half of beaten eggs into the skillet and coat the bottom of the pan. When egg mixture has partially set, scrape the edges and tip the pan so that uncooked egg mixture at the top can spread to the hot cooking surface of the skillet.

5. Immediately after, add half of vegetable mixture and ham to half of the omelet and continue to cook until egg mixture is almost fully set.

6. Using a spatula, fold the empty half over top of the ham and veggies. Cook for 2 minutes longer, then serve.

7. Repeat the process with the remaining 2 eggs and remaining half of vegetable mixture and ham to make the second omelet.

8. Transfer to plate, season with sea salt and pepper, and serve hot.

**PALEO COMPASS**

This is a diverse omelet that you can add any leftover proteins from the fridge into, as well as any leftover vegetables. In this case, make sure the proteins and vegetables are balanced to give you energy throughout your entire morning.

# Sweet Breakfasts

## In This Chapter

- Kick-start your day with pancakes, crêpes, and more
- Oatmeal without the oats
- Using Paleo-friendly flours in traditional breakfast recipes
- Protein-packed muffins that satisfy any sweet tooth

The Paleo way of eating helps you lose weight and regain your health partly by removing those typical Western, high-glycemic foods from your diet. But that doesn't mean sweet foods like pancakes and muffins are out of the question! They can be made with nut flours and fruit, instead of refined flours and caustic sugars to keep your blood sugar relatively stable. While it's best to combine the sweeter breakfasts with a rich protein source like meat or eggs, they can be eaten on their own every so often, too.

The sweet breakfast recipes in this chapter will widen your breakfast horizons and let you indulge your sweet tooth once in a while. With the following recipes, you can move beyond the typical sugary breakfasts to foods that will truly nourish you for the whole day.

# Almond Flour Pancakes

A lightly sweet take on the original, these delicious pancakes are a bit nutty, with hints of coconut and applesauce.

| Yield: | Prep time: | Cook time: | Serving size: |
|---|---|---|---|
| 6 pancakes | 10 minutes | 15 minutes | 3 pancakes |
| **Each serving has:** | | | |
| 550 calories | 22 g carbohydrates | 47 g fat | 19 g protein |

1 cup almond flour

½ cup unsweetened applesauce

1 TB. coconut flour

2 medium eggs

¼ cup water (or use soda water for slightly fluffier pancakes)

¼ tsp. whole nutmeg, freshly grated

¼ tsp. sea salt

3 tsp. coconut oil

1 cup fresh berries

1. Combine almond flour, applesauce, coconut flour, eggs, water, nutmeg, and sea salt in a bowl, and mix together completely with a fork. Batter will appear a little thicker than usual pancake mix.

2. Heat a nonstick frying pan over medium heat with 1 teaspoon coconut oil.

3. Drop ¼ cup batter onto the hot pan. Spread out batter slightly if desired.

4. Flip like a normal pancake when the bubbles start showing up on the top, and cook for 1 to 2 more minutes.

5. Add more coconut oil to the pan and repeat with remaining batter.

6. Top with fresh berries and serve.

**PALEO COMPASS**

These are very dense and protein-rich pancakes, so you probably won't need as many as their typical carb-loaded, grain-based counterparts to feel full. Also, when cooking, give them plenty of space in the pan or griddle so you can properly flip them. They don't stick together like a standard pancake, so you have to be a bit more careful.

# No-Oat "Oatmeal"

This hearty and dense nonoatmeal blends ginger, bananas, pumpkin seeds, and other nuts to fully engage the palette.

| Yield: | Prep time: | Cook time: | Serving size: |
|---|---|---|---|
| 3 cups | 5 minutes | 15 minutes | 1½ cups |
| **Each serving has:** | | | |
| 448 calories | 21 g carbohydrates | 34 g fat | 18 g protein |

¼ cup walnuts

¼ cup pecans

2 TB. ground flaxseed

1 tsp. ground cinnamon

¼ tsp. whole nutmeg, freshly grated

¼ tsp. ground ginger

3 medium eggs

¼ cup unsweetened almond milk

1 banana, mashed

1 TB. almond butter

2 tsp. pumpkin seeds

1 cup blueberries

1. Add walnuts, pecans, flaxseed, cinnamon, nutmeg, and ginger to a food processor and pulse mixture to a coarse grain (make sure to stop before it is ground into a powder). Set aside.

2. Whisk together eggs and almond milk until consistency thickens and becomes loose custard.

3. Thoroughly blend mashed banana and almond butter together and add it to custard, mixing well.

4. Stir in coarse nut mixture.

5. In a medium saucepan, warm mixture on the stove until it reaches the desired consistency; this should only take a few minutes. Stir frequently.

6. To serve, spoon into a bowl and sprinkle pumpkin seeds and blueberries on top. Add more almond milk if desired.

**Variation:** If cinnamon, nutmeg, and ginger aren't your thing, you can easily change the flavor profile of this dish by adding several different types of berries or a bit of raw honey.

# Almost Oatmeal

Few things really bring out the flavor of apples better than cinnamon and freshly grated nutmeg. These spices also provide a warm complement to the nuttiness of the almond butter.

| Yield: | Prep time: | Cook time: | Serving size: |
| --- | --- | --- | --- |
| 4 cups | 5 minutes | 5 minutes | 2 cups |
| **Each serving has:** | | | |
| 669 calories | 59 g carbohydrates | 44 g fat | 16 g protein |

3 cups unsweetened applesauce

8 TB. raw, chunky almond butter

5 TB. raw, unsweetened canned coconut milk

½ tsp. cinnamon

¼ tsp. whole nutmeg, freshly grated

1. Combine applesauce, almond butter, and coconut milk in a small pan over medium heat, stirring often.

2. Spoon into a bowl.

3. Sprinkle cinnamon and nutmeg on top and serve.

**Variation:** Like regular oatmeal, there are many ways to customize this dish—add fresh berries and nuts, or substitute almond milk for coconut milk. It's a good standby recipe, and the diversity of the toppings keep it from becoming boring.

# Banana Almond Pancakes

With lots of fresh fruit, these pancakes are naturally sweet, making them a great choice for kids who are used to eating sugary breakfast cereal. The blueberries help soften the banana flavor, and the nuts and almond butter provide a protein-packed base.

| Yield: | Prep time: | Cook time: | | Serving size: |
|---|---|---|---|---|
| 6 pancakes | 5 minutes | 20 minutes | | 3 pancakes |
| **Each serving has:** | | | | |
| 664 calories | 46 g carbohydrates | 48 g fat | | 17 g protein |

| | |
|---|---|
| 4 bananas, mashed | 2 TB. coconut oil |
| 2 medium eggs | 2 cups fresh blueberries |
| 5 TB. almond butter | ½ cup walnuts, chopped |

1. Combine mashed bananas, eggs, and almond butter and whisk until well blended.

2. Heat a nonstick skillet over medium-low heat, and add coconut oil when pan is hot. Note: pancakes will stick to griddle and be difficult to turn if heat is too high.

3. Pour small discs of batter onto the hot pan.

4. Add blueberries and walnuts as pancakes cook on one side. Flip when batter loses its "tackiness" around the edges and begins to bubble.

5. Cook other side slowly over medium-low heat until fully cooked.

6. Transfer to plate and eat hot.

**Variation:** Take advantage of whatever fruit is in season to garnish these pancakes and help keep weekly grocery costs down. You can also boil the blueberries in a pot with a little water until the berries burst, creating a delicious berry syrup.

# Breakfast Smoothie

This quick and tasty drink is bursting with blueberry and strawberry flavor.

| Yield: | Prep time: | Cook time: | Serving size: |
|---|---|---|---|
| 4 cups | 5 minutes | 3 minutes | 2 cups |
| **Each serving has:** | | | |
| 238 calories | 24 g carbohydrates | 19 g fat | 3 g protein |

1 cup frozen strawberries

1 cup frozen blueberries

⅔ cup unsweetened shredded coconut

1 cup almond milk

2 eggs (safest if from pastured chickens)

1. Fill a blender with strawberries and blueberries and quickly pulse with 2 ounces hot water to break them up.

2. Add shredded coconut, almond milk, and eggs.

3. Continue to blend until smooth, then pour into 2 glasses and serve.

**Variation:** Feel free to leave out eggs if you want a sweeter smoothie, or if you can't get pastured eggs and are cautious.

**PALEO COMPASS**

This is a very fast breakfast that can help you get out the door when you're running behind. It doesn't have a lot of protein, though, so consider bringing along a hard-boiled egg or some deli meat in a pinch for a complete breakfast on the go.

# Paleo Pumpkin Muffins

These muffins have no added sugar, and only 4 tablespoons of honey make them delicately sweet with a rich pumpkin pie flavor.

| Yield: | Prep time: | Cook time: | Serving size: |
|---|---|---|---|
| 6 muffins | 15 minutes | 25 minutes | 2 muffins |
| **Each serving has:** | | | |
| 652 calories | 46 g carbohydrates | 44 g fat | 24 g protein |

½ tsp. coconut oil

1½ cups almond flour

¾ cup canned pumpkin

3 large eggs

1 tsp. baking powder

1 tsp. baking soda

½ tsp. ground cinnamon

1½ tsp. pumpkin pie spice

⅛ tsp. salt

4 TB. raw honey

2 tsp. almond butter

30 whole almonds

1. Preheat the oven to 350°F.

2. Coat 6 muffin cups with coconut oil (or use paper liners and add about ½ teaspoon melted coconut oil to batter).

3. Mix almond flour, pumpkin, eggs, baking powder, baking soda, cinnamon, pumpkin pie spice, salt, honey, and almond butter. Pour batter into the muffin cups.

4. Bake at 350°F for 25 minutes on the middle rack.

5. Lightly press five almonds into the top of each muffin right after you take them out of the oven.

6. Let cool before removing from pan. Serve warm or cold.

**Variation:** Substitute the canned pumpkin with summer squash or fresh pumpkin. You'll want to bake it until soft, and process it in a food processor until it's thick and smooth.

# Tapioca Crêpes

These slightly sweet crêpes, filled with almond butter and blueberries, are a light and airy mouthful.

| Yield: | Prep time: | Cook time: | Serving size: |
|---|---|---|---|
| 2 crêpes | 5 minutes | 10 minutes | 1 crêpe |
| **Each serving has:** | | | |
| 607 calories | 69 g carbohydrates | 32 g fat | 10 g protein |

1 cup tapioca flour (or tapioca starch)

1 cup raw unsweetened canned coconut milk

1 large egg

1 TB. coconut oil

2 TB. almond butter

½ cup blueberries

1. Combine tapioca flour, coconut milk, and egg in a medium bowl.

2. Heat a nonstick skillet over medium heat and add coconut oil when pan is hot.

3. When hot, pour in about ⅓ cup of mixture and tilt the pan in all directions to spread out the batter.

4. Cook both sides until very lightly browned (2 to 3 minutes each side).

5. Top with almond butter and blueberries and serve.

**Variation:** You can put anything in these crêpes that you can imagine—applesauce and cinnamon, sautéed vegetables, almond butter and blueberries, or crumbled bacon. Experiment with seasonal berries in the summer and savory vegetables or warm spices in the winter.

# Carrot Banana Muffins

The carrots in this dish are surprisingly sweet. When paired with the bananas, these muffins are sure to satisfy even the most discerning sweet tooth.

| Yield: | Prep time: | Cook time: | Serving size: |
|---|---|---|---|
| 12 muffins | 15 minutes | 25 minutes | 2 muffins |
| **Each serving has:** | | | |
| 288 calories | 24 g carbohydrates | 20 g fat | 8 g protein |

2 cups almond flour

2 tsp. baking soda

1 tsp. sea salt

1 TB. cinnamon

1 cup dates, pitted

3 ripe bananas

3 medium eggs

1 tsp. apple cider vinegar

¼ cup coconut oil

1½ cups carrots, shredded

¾ cup walnuts, finely chopped

1. Preheat oven to 350°F.

2. In a small bowl, combine almond flour, baking soda, sea salt, and cinnamon. Set aside.

3. In a food processor, combine dates, bananas, eggs, apple cider vinegar, and coconut oil.

4. Transfer both mixtures to a large bowl and blend until completely combined.

5. Fold in carrots and walnuts.

6. Spoon mixture into the paper-lined muffin tins. Note: you can also lightly grease the muffin tins with coconut oil instead of using paper liners.

7. Bake at 350°F for 25 minutes.

8. Let cool before removing from pan. Serve warm or cold.

**PALEO COMPASS**

These delicious muffins keep well when frozen, so it's easy to make a large batch when you have extra time. They thaw quickly and make a great traveling snack or breakfast on the go.

# Satisfying Snacks and Salads

## In This Chapter

- Light grab-and-go snacks
- Filling favorites
- Paleo twists on traditional snacks
- Candy bars, Paleo style

A common myth is that snacking is bad for your health. The truth is that snacking itself isn't bad for you—it's just the foods you choose to munch on that can cause problems. Grazing on candy, chips, soda, pastries, and other high-glycemic, omega-6-laced foods is pretty bad for you. It can lead to weight gain and inflammation. However, eating enough of the right foods throughout the day, like the snacks and salads in this chapter, can actually be *helpful* for blood sugar balance and weight loss. We included salads in this chapter because they can be light enough to be just snacks, or filling enough to be stand-alone meals.

We've arranged this chapter from lightest to most filling dishes. All of them are deliciously Paleo.

# Berries with Balsamic Vinegar and Almonds

This surprising combination offers the sweetness that you crave, with the protein that will keep you going.

| Yield: | Prep time: | Serving size: | |
|---|---|---|---|
| 2 cups | 5 minutes | 1 cup | |
| **Each serving has:** | | | |
| 207 calories | 29 g carbohydrates | 11 g fat | 5 g protein |

1 to 2 cups fresh berries

4 tsp. balsamic vinegar

⅓ cup slivered almonds

1. Wash and slice fresh berries (if needed).

2. Evenly separate berries between two small bowls.

3. Sprinkle 2 teaspoons balsamic vinegar over each serving.

4. Top with slivered almonds and serve.

**Variation:** For an even sweeter treat, replace balsamic vinegar with 1 tablespoon raw honey and add ⅓ cup chopped macadamia nuts.

# Cantaloupe and Avocado Salad with Honey-Lime Dressing

This sweet salad is excellent in late summer, when cantaloupe and tomatoes are at their best in most regions.

| Yield: | Prep time: | Serving size: | |
| --- | --- | --- | --- |
| 4 cups | 15 minutes | 1 cup | |
| **Each serving has:** | | | |
| 192 calories | 22 g carbohydrates | 13 g fat | 3 g protein |

| | |
| --- | --- |
| 3 TB. fresh lime juice | 1 (3-lb.) cantaloupe, quartered and seeded |
| 4 tsp. raw honey | |
| 2 TB. olive oil | 1 avocado |
| ½ tsp. coarse sea salt | 1 cup cherry or grape tomatoes, halved |

1. In a large bowl, whisk together lime juice, honey, olive oil, and sea salt. Set aside.

2. Cut each cantaloupe quarter in half lengthwise. Run a knife between flesh and skin of melon; discard skin. Slice each wedge lengthwise into ½-inch pieces.

3. Cut avocado in quarters lengthwise and then into ½-inch-thick slices. Add cantaloupe, avocado, and grape tomatoes to a bowl with dressing and toss to coat. Serve.

# Fruit Salad with Cinnamon

A simple rendition of a classic salad with plenty of flavor.

| Yield: | Prep time: | Serving size: | |
|---|---|---|---|
| 2 cups | 15 minutes | 1 cup | |
| **Each serving has:** | | | |
| 224 calories | 23 g carbohydrates | 15 g fat | 5 g protein |

1 orange, peeled and diced

1 apple, diced

½ cup pecans or walnuts, chopped (optional)

½ tsp. cinnamon

1. Place orange and apple into two bowls.

2. Sprinkle with chopped pecans (if using) and/or cinnamon and serve.

**PALEO COMPASS**

If you make this recipe ahead of time, sprinkle the chopped apple with lemon juice to keep it from turning brown.

# Guacamole Deviled Eggs

So good, you may never go back to the original!

| Yield: | Prep time: | Cook time: | Serving size: |
|---|---|---|---|
| 8 deviled egg halves | 10 minutes | 15 minutes | 2 deviled egg halves |

| Each serving has: | | | |
|---|---|---|---|
| 166 calories | 4 g carbohydrates | 12 g fat | 11 g protein |

4 eggs, hard-boiled

1 avocado

2 tsp. hot sauce

1 tsp. lemon juice

Sea salt

Freshly ground black pepper

4 thin slices smoked beef, cut in half

1. Peel hard-boiled eggs and cut in half. Spoon out yolks into a small bowl.

2. Mash yolks with avocado, hot sauce, and lemon juice. Season to taste with sea salt and pepper.

3. Refill egg whites with yolk mixture.

4. Top with smoked beef slices and serve.

# Orange, Avocado, and Cashew Salad

This fresh and juicy salad is a quick treat that provides sweet and salty flavors. It's a perfect solution for most cravings.

| Yield: | Prep time: | Serving size: | |
|---|---|---|---|
| 3 cups | 10 minutes | 1½ cups | |
| **Each serving has:** | | | |
| 306 calories | 25 g carbohydrates | 25 g fat | 4 g protein |

1 large orange

2 handfuls spinach, arugula, or watercress

1 large ripe avocado, diced

¼ cup cashews

1 TB. olive oil

Sea salt

Freshly ground black pepper

1. Prepare orange by cutting off rind and outer membrane and slicing out wedges of fruit between segments. Do this over a bowl and set remaining juice aside.

2. Divide spinach between two plates and top with orange segments, avocado, and cashews.

3. Add a drizzle of olive oil and any juice left over from oranges. Season to taste with sea salt and pepper and serve.

**Variation:** Add cooked chicken breast to each salad to make this a more filling and complete lunch or dinner.

# Salsa Salad

This lively salad showcases the best parts of fresh salsa. Juicy Roma tomatoes, spicy pepper, rich avocado, and fresh cilantro combine for an unbeatable flavor combination.

| Yield: | Prep time: | Serving size: | |
|---|---|---|---|
| 3 cups | 15 minutes | 1½ cups | |
| **Each serving has:** | | | |
| 326 calories | 31 g carbohydrates | 22 g fat | 5 g protein |

1 bunch cilantro, chopped

4 Roma tomatoes, diced

¼ small red onion, finely diced

1 small chili pepper, finely diced

Handful whole dulse leaf, torn into
    bite-size pieces

1 TB. olive oil

¼ tsp. sea salt

1 medium avocado, diced

1. Toss cilantro, Roma tomatoes, red onion, chili pepper, and dulse leaf together in a large bowl.

2. Add olive oil and sea salt and toss again lightly.

3. Split between two bowls.

4. Top with diced avocado and serve.

**PALEO COMPASS**

Dulse leaf is a dried sea vegetable rich in calcium, magnesium, iron, and many vitamins. It can be found it most natural food stores, or can be easily ordered online.

# Spicy Tuna Salad

This salad is tart, salty, and spicy—the trifecta when paired with the rich taste of tuna.

| Yield: | Prep time: | Serving size: | |
|---|---|---|---|
| 2 salads | 5 minutes | 1 salad | |
| **Each serving has:** | | | |
| 413 calories | 30 g carbohydrates | 22 g fat | 29 g protein |

2 (6-oz.) cans oil-packed tuna, drained

1 cup green olives, chopped

2 green onions, chopped

1 jalapeño pepper, finely chopped, seeds removed

3 TB. capers, rinsed

2 TB. red chili flakes

1 head butter lettuce or mixed greens

1 tsp. olive oil

Juice of 3 lemons

1 avocado, sliced

1. Combine tuna, green olives, green onions, jalapeño pepper, capers, and red chili flakes in a large bowl.

2. Spoon onto a bed of lettuce and drizzle with olive oil and fresh lemon juice. Top with sliced avocado and serve.

**PALEO COMPASS**

Let the flavors of the tuna, olives, onions, jalapeño pepper, capers, and chili flakes meld overnight for a better tasting salad. Be sure to wait until the last minute to spoon the mixture on top of the butter lettuce so that the lettuce stays crisp.

# Sautéed Shrimp

This recipe is perfect for days when you don't have much time to cook but crave something warm to snack on.

| Yield: | Prep time: | Cook time: | Serving size: |
|---|---|---|---|
| 2 cups | 5 minutes | 20 minutes | 1 cup |
| **Each serving has:** | | | |
| 297 calories | 7 g carbohydrates | 19 g fat | 147 g protein |

2 TB. olive oil

½ lb. raw shrimp, deveined and peeled

2 TB. chili powder

1 TB. garlic powder

½ TB. parsley

Cayenne pepper

Freshly ground black pepper

1. Heat olive oil in a sauté pan.

2. Once hot, add shrimp and sauté until just pink.

3. Add chili powder, garlic powder, and parsley. Season to taste with cayenne pepper and black pepper.

4. Continue to sauté for 7 to 10 minutes or until cooked through.

5. Transfer to a plate and serve hot.

# Spinach Salad

This tangy salad has just the right amount of zing to be an excellent accompaniment to fish.

| Yield: | Prep time: | Serving size: | |
| --- | --- | --- | --- |
| 4 cups | 15 minutes | 2 cups | |
| **Each serving has:** | | | |
| 142 calories | 5 g carbohydrates | 14 g fat | 1 g protein |

4 cups fresh spinach

4 green onions, chopped

Juice of 1 lemon

2 TB. olive oil

¼ tsp. freshly ground black pepper

1. Wash spinach well, drain, and chop.

2. Let chopped spinach sit for a few minutes and then squeeze out excess water.

3. Put spinach in a medium bowl and add green onions, lemon juice, olive oil, and pepper.

4. Toss and serve.

**Variation:** For a fresh take on this recipe, use red onion instead of green onions, and substitute fresh orange juice for lemon juice. Top with toasted almonds for more protein and healthy fat.

# Watermelon Freeze

This refreshing snack is perfect for a summertime blood sugar boost!

| Yield: | Prep time: | Cook time: | Serving size: |
|---|---|---|---|
| 6 cups | 20 minutes | 4 hours | ½ cup |

| Each serving has: | | | |
|---|---|---|---|
| 30 calories | 6 g carbohydrates | 0 g fat | 1 g protein |

4 cups watermelon, seeded and cubed

2 cups cantaloupe, cubed

3 fresh mint leaves or 1 mint tea bag

1 cup water

Juice of 1 lemon

Paper muffin liners or small paper cups

12 flat wooden sticks

1. Purée watermelon and cantaloupe in a food processor until smooth.

2. Place melon mixture in a medium saucepan over medium heat and bring to a simmer. Cook for 15 minutes.

3. Meanwhile, in another pan, steep mint leaves in water for about 3 minutes.

4. Strain and add this infusion to cooked melons.

5. Turn off heat and stir in lemon juice.

6. Line a muffin pan with paper muffin liners (may instead use small paper cups or ice cube trays).

7. Pour melon purée into each liner and freeze.

8. When mixture begins to firm up, insert flat wooden sticks into the center of each.

9. Freeze until completely hard or the papers will not peel easily away.

10. Remove papers before serving.

**Variation:** This recipe can easily be made into a smoothie. Chill melon purée, and blend with ½ cup to 1 cup ice in the blender. Makes about 4 smoothies.

# Basil Spinach Chicken Salad

The unmatched flavor of fresh basil shines in this beautiful summertime salad.

| Yield: | Prep time: | Cook time: | Serving size: |
|---|---|---|---|
| 6 cups | 5 minutes | 5 minutes | 3 cups |

| Each serving has: | | | |
|---|---|---|---|
| 490 calories | 15 g carbohydrates | 20 g fat | 59 g protein |

2 TB. coconut oil

12 oz. chicken breast, cut into narrow strips

½ medium yellow onion, diced

2 medium tomatoes, diced

4 cups fresh spinach, rinsed and patted dry

10 sprigs fresh basil, rinsed

1. Heat a small skillet over medium-high heat. Add coconut oil when hot. Cook chicken strips until they start to brown on all sides and are fully cooked throughout. Set aside.

2. Add yellow onion and sauté until soft and translucent. Add tomatoes and cook for 1 to 2 more minutes.

3. Add spinach and basil to the pan and cook for 1 minute.

4. Arrange chicken strips on top and serve immediately.

**Variation:** For a meal on the go, combine all vegetables while still raw and serve cold with olive oil, balsamic vinegar, and precooked chicken.

# Chef Salad

This take on a classic salad leaves nothing to be desired—sweet tomatoes, crunchy celery, salty bacon, and the tang of fresh lemon.

| Yield: | Prep time: | Cook time: | Serving size: |
|---|---|---|---|
| 4 cups | 15 minutes | 10 minutes | 2 cups |

| Each serving has: | | | |
|---|---|---|---|
| 521 calories | 20 g carbohydrates | 30 g fat | 39 g protein |

1 head red leaf lettuce, rinsed and chopped

8 cherry tomatoes, halved

4 green onions, sliced thin

2 stalks celery, diced

1 avocado, diced

4 medium eggs, hard-boiled, shelled, and halved

2 slices bacon, cooked and crumbled

8 oz. ham, diced

2 tsp. olive oil

Juice of 1 lemon

1. Divide red leaf lettuce between two plates.

2. Top each plate with cherry tomatoes, green onions, celery, avocado, eggs, bacon, and ham.

3. Drizzle with olive oil and fresh lemon juice and serve cold.

**PALEO COMPASS**

Much of this recipe can be prepared ahead of time. Cook the bacon, hard-boil the eggs, and prepare the vegetables the night before to make assembly easy. Just don't dice the avocado beforehand or it will turn brown.

# Chicken Fajita Salad

Coconut oil is the perfect complement to this warm fajita mix, especially when served over crisp lettuce and sweet bell peppers.

| Yield: | Prep time: | Cook time: | Serving size: |
| --- | --- | --- | --- |
| 16 cups | 10 minutes | 20 minutes | 4 cups |
| **Each serving has:** | | | |
| 425 calories | 35 g carbohydrates | 21 g fat | 29 g protein |

2 TB. coconut oil

1 medium yellow onion, diced

1 lb. boneless, skinless chicken breasts, cut into ½-in. slices

1 tsp. ground cumin

3 tsp. dried oregano

½ tsp. sea salt

2 large green bell peppers, chopped

2 large heads red leaf lettuce, rinsed and shredded

4 medium tomatoes, diced

2 avocados, sliced

1. Heat a skillet over medium-high heat. When hot, add coconut oil and yellow onion. Sauté until onion pieces are soft and slightly translucent.

2. Add chicken, cumin, oregano, and sea salt to the onions and continue to cook, stirring often.

3. When chicken has browned, add green bell peppers and cook until tender.

4. Divide red leaf lettuce between two plates.

5. Top each plate with chicken fajita mix, tomatoes, and avocados and serve hot.

**PALEO COMPASS**

If you are packing this lunch for work, keep the warm fajita mix in a separate container from the rest of the salad and add it when you are ready to eat, to keep the lettuce crisp. It's worth warming up at the office so the flavors can really shine.

# Paleo Trail Mix

Feel free to mix it up a bit and add the dried fruit and nuts you like most.

| Yield: | Prep time: | Serving size: | |
|---|---|---|---|
| 4 cups | 10 minutes | 1 cup | |
| **Each serving has:** | | | |
| 496 calories | 44 g carbohydrates | 33 g fat | 16 g protein |

1 cup whole almonds
½ cup whole cashews
½ cup raw pumpkin seeds
½ cup raw sunflower seeds

½ cup raisins (golden raisins suggested)
½ cup dried currants
½ cup dried blueberries

1. Combine almonds, cashews, pumpkin seeds, sunflower seeds, raisins, currants, and blueberries.

2. Store in an airtight container until ready to serve, or serve immediately.

**Variation:** It's easy to change this recipe to fit your preferences. Add ½ cup carob chips, and replace currants with ½ cup dried cherries for another satisfying version. Look for dried fruits without any added sugar.

# Paleo Candy Bars

These are so tasty that you'll have to be careful not to eat them all at once! This high-calorie snack is perfect for something sweet to bring on your next backpacking trip.

| Yield: | Prep time: | Cook time: | Serving size: |
|---|---|---|---|
| 4 2×2-in. bars | 15 minutes | 10 minutes | 1 2×2-in. bar |

| Each serving has: | | | |
|---|---|---|---|
| 301 calories | 13 g carbohydrates | 28 g fat | 6 g protein |

| | |
|---|---|
| 1 TB. raw honey (optional; add more to taste) | ½ cup ground nuts such as almonds or hazelnuts |
| 3 TB. coconut oil | ¾ cup unsweetened shredded coconut |
| ¼ cup carob powder or cocoa (optional) | Parchment paper |

1. Melt honey (if using) and coconut oil in a saucepan over medium heat.

2. Once combined, add carob powder (if using), ground nuts, and shredded coconut and mix together.

3. Pour mixture onto a small baking sheet covered in parchment paper. Form into a square when cool enough to touch.

4. Refrigerate until hardened (approximately 2 hours). Cut into four servings and serve chilled or at room temperature.

> **PALEO COMPASS**
>
> The nuts should be ground to a meal-like consistency. You can grind them yourself in a food processor, or buy ground nuts.

# Paleo Niçoise Salad

Between the cherry tomatoes, lemon, and spices, this salad is anything but dull, and the capers add a bit of sourness.

| Yield: | Prep time: | Cook time: | Serving size: |
|---|---|---|---|
| 6 cups | 15 minutes | 15 minutes | 3 cups |

| Each serving has: | | | |
|---|---|---|---|
| 638 calories | 17 g carbohydrates | 37 g fat | 61 g protein |

2 TB. olive oil

Juice of 1 lemon

¼ tsp. sea salt

¼ tsp. freshly ground black pepper

1 large head butter lettuce, shredded

Handful (10 to 12) green beans, chopped into 2-in. pieces

1 cup cherry tomatoes

2 TB. capers, rinsed

2 (6-oz.) cans oil-packed tuna, drained

4 hard-boiled eggs, shelled and halved

½ cup kalamata olives, pitted

1. Whisk olive oil, lemon juice, sea salt, and pepper together in a small bowl.

2. Toss butter lettuce, green beans, cherry tomatoes, and capers with olive oil mixture to coat.

3. Top with tuna, eggs, and kalamata olives to serve.

# PB & J Paleo Style

This easy snack is deceptively satisfying.

| Yield: | Prep time: | Serving size: | |
|---|---|---|---|
| 1½ cups | 5 minutes | ¾ cup | |
| **Each serving has:** | | | |
| 420 calories | 27 g carbohydrates | 33 g fat | 13 g protein |

1 cup fresh or frozen blueberries          4 TB. unsweetened almond butter
(or other berries of choice)

1. Divide blueberries between two bowls.

2. Add 2 tablespoons almond butter to each bowl and mix. Serve.

# Raw Cabbage and Pineapple Salad

This simple salad is sweet and nutty. The vibrant colors of the cabbage and pineapple also make it an attractive dish to serve a crowd.

| Yield: | Prep time: | Serving size: | |
|---|---|---|---|
| 2 salads | 5 minutes | 1 salad | |
| **Each serving has:** | | | |
| 396 calories | 24 g carbohydrates | 31 g fat | 10 g protein |

½ head red cabbage, shredded          2 TB. olive oil (optional)
½ small pineapple, diced               1 cup hazelnuts, chopped

1. Combine cabbage and pineapple. Drizzle with olive oil (if using).

2. Store salad up to 3 days. Top with hazelnuts right before serving.

**PALEO COMPASS**

This salad keeps really well in the refrigerator if the hazelnuts are left out. Just remember to add them right before serving to get the important fats and protein.

# Appetizers, Sides, and Condiments

## In This Chapter

- Side dishes and appetizers that feature fresh veggies
- A savory spin on watermelon
- Using Paleo ingredients to update old favorites
- Tasty condiments to keep on hand

You may be surprised to find that some of your old favorite side dishes, appetizers, and condiments are naturally Paleo friendly. Guacamole is usually just avocados, lime juice, and veggies, all of which are Paleo. Sometimes it just takes changing one ingredient to make something Paleo, like the kind of mayo you use to make coleslaw or the dipping sauce in shrimp cocktail. Some of the recipes in this chapter switch out integral ingredients in classic recipes to make them Paleo, while keeping the essence of the old favorite intact, like the Cauliflower Rice recipe.

The recipes on the following pages are incredible additions to entrées, and the appetizers are enticing dinner party conversation starters. Use them to make your plate more colorful and nutrient dense, and to add more complex flavors to the mix. And, of course, to impress your non-Paleo friends!

# Apple Coleslaw

This fresh and light coleslaw has just the right amount of zip.

| Yield: | Prep time: | Serving size: | |
|---|---|---|---|
| 4 cups | 15 minutes | 1 cup | |
| **Each serving has:** | | | |
| 213 calories | 24 g carbohydrates | 14 g fat | 2 g protein |

½ small red or green cabbage, chopped

1 tart apple (Granny Smith recommended), grated or chopped

1 large stalk celery, chopped

1 medium green bell pepper, chopped

¼ cup olive oil

Juice of 1 lemon

2 TB. raw honey

1. Toss red cabbage, apple, celery, and green bell pepper together in a large bowl.

2. In a smaller bowl, whisk together olive oil, lemon juice, and honey.

3. Drizzle olive oil mixture over coleslaw and toss to coat.

4. Serve cold. Refrigerate overnight for more flavor.

# Butternut Squash with Cranberries

The warm spices in this lunch keep you toasty on a cold day. The tangy cranberries pair nicely with the velvety cream of the rich coconut milk.

| Yield: | Prep time: | Cook time: | Serving size: |
|---|---|---|---|
| 2 cups | 10 minutes | 15 minutes | 1 cup |
| **Each serving has:** | | | |
| 218 calories | 25 g carbohydrates | 14 g fat | 2 g protein |

1 cup butternut squash, peeled
  and diced

½ medium white onion, diced

2 cloves garlic, sliced

1 tsp. coconut oil

1 cup dried cranberries

1 (6-oz.) can coconut milk

1 tsp. curry powder

1 tsp. cinnamon

1. Place butternut squash on a cookie sheet and bake at 425°F for 15 minutes or until tender.

2. In a medium frying pan on high heat, sauté white onion and garlic in coconut oil for 1 to 2 minutes.

3. Add cooked squash and cook 2 or 3 minutes.

4. Add cranberries, coconut milk, curry powder, and cinnamon, and stir frequently until milk is heated. Serve hot.

**PALEO COMPASS**

This lunch is best paired with a lean protein. Add a sliced chicken breast on top or bake a filet of white fish to serve alongside.

# Cauliflower Rice

Similar to traditional rice, this dish absorbs the flavors of whatever you serve it with. It's slightly nutty and a perfect complement to curry and stir-fry dishes.

| Yield: | Prep time: | Cooking time: | Serving size: |
|---|---|---|---|
| 4 cups | 10 minutes | 10 minutes | 1 cup |

| Each serving has: | | | |
|---|---|---|---|
| 66 calories | 8 g carbohydrates | 4 g fat | 3 g protein |

| | |
|---|---|
| 1 medium-size head cauliflower | 1 TB. coconut oil |

1. Wash cauliflower and remove florets from stem; discard stem.

2. Rough-chop florets.

3. Heat a large skillet over medium-high heat. Add coconut oil when pan is hot.

4. Add cauliflower and cook until slightly tender.

5. Remove from heat. Place cauliflower in a food processor, along with any desired seasonings.

6. Pulse until cauliflower has a grainy, ricelike consistency. Serve warm or cold.

**Variation:** Experiment with optional seasonings (sea salt, granulated garlic, ginger, cayenne, coconut aminos, curry powder, or freshly ground black pepper) to help complement whatever dish you're serving Cauliflower Rice with.

# Chard and Cashew Sauté

This is a flavorful way to incorporate more dark leafy greens into your diet.

| Yield: | Prep time: | Cook time: | Serving size: |
|---|---|---|---|
| 2 cups | 5 minutes | 10 minutes | 1 cup |
| **Each serving has:** | | | |
| 217 calories | 10 g carbohydrates | 19 g fat | 6 g protein |

1 bunch Swiss chard

1 TB. coconut or olive oil

½ cup cashews

Sea salt

Freshly ground black pepper

1. Wash Swiss chard and remove tough stems. Chop Swiss chard into thin strips.

2. Heat a large skillet over medium heat, and add coconut oil when the pan is hot.

3. Add Swiss chard to the hot skillet, along with cashews.

4. Sauté, tossing occasionally, until Swiss chard leaves just begin to wilt.

5. Season to taste with sea salt and pepper. Serve warm.

**Variation:** For a real southern-style recipe, replace coconut or olive oil with ¼ cup bacon drippings, and add a dash of cayenne pepper.

# Endive Salmon Poppers

Crisp endive and potent red onion cut through the rich smoked salmon to create a harmony of flavor in each bite.

| Yield: | Prep time: | Serving size: | |
| --- | --- | --- | --- |
| 10 poppers | 10 minutes | 5 poppers | |
| **Each serving has:** | | | |
| 312 calories | 13 g carbohydrates | 20 g fat | 24 g protein |

1 to 2 heads endive

4 oz. smoked salmon, sliced

¼ red onion, minced

½ medium avocado, sliced

Sea salt

Freshly ground black pepper

2 tsp. olive oil

1. Wash and separate endive leaves.

2. Top each leaf with smoked salmon, red onion, and avocado.

3. Season to taste with sea salt and pepper, and drizzle with olive oil. Serve cold.

**PALEO COMPASS**

These showy poppers make a great party appetizer. The endive is sturdy enough to hold up when made a few hours ahead of time. If making ahead of time, substitute capers for the avocado, which turns brown quickly. If you can't find endive at the store, look for romaine lettuce hearts.

# Fresh Tomatoes with Basil

The slightly peppery and sweet taste of basil mixes with the tartness of the tomatoes and the sea salt to make this simple dish come alive with flavor.

| Yield: | Prep time: | Serving size: | |
| --- | --- | --- | --- |
| 2 cups | 10 minutes | 1 cup | |
| **Each serving has:** | | | |
| 153 calories | 6 g carbohydrates | 14 g fat | 0 g protein |

1 pint cherry or grape tomatoes, sliced in half

Several sprigs of fresh basil, finely chopped

1 TB. balsamic vinegar

2 TB. olive oil

Sea salt

1. Place cherry tomatoes in a bowl and sprinkle with basil. Drizzle with balsamic vinegar and olive oil.

2. Season to taste with sea salt and serve.

# Roasted Asparagus

This easy side dish goes with just about anything.

| Yield: | Prep time: | Cook time: | Serving size: |
| --- | --- | --- | --- |
| 20 spears | 5 minutes | 25 minutes | 5 spears |
| **Each serving has:** | | | |
| 52 calories | 5 g carbohydrates | 4 g fat | 2 g protein |

1 large bunch asparagus (about 20 spears)

1 TB. olive oil

2 tsp. dried thyme

Sea salt

Freshly ground black pepper

1. Preheat oven to 400°F.

2. Wash and remove tough ends of asparagus.

3. Place asparagus in a roasting pan or on a baking sheet.

4. Drizzle olive oil over asparagus and sprinkle with thyme. Toss together until well coated.

5. Bake for 10 minutes, then reduce the heat to 250°F and bake for 15 more minutes or until tender.

6. Season to taste with sea salt and pepper. Serve hot.

**PALEO COMPASS**

Try this recipe on the grill! Follow steps 1 through 4 and then add a dash of sea salt and pepper. Grill in a basket for 5 to 8 minutes, then serve.

# Roasted Beets with Balsamic Glaze

This is a robust and earthy combination of flavors.

| Yield: | Prep time: | Cook time: | Serving size: |
|---|---|---|---|
| 4 cups | 10 minutes | 60 minutes | 1 cup |

| **Each serving has:** | | | |
|---|---|---|---|
| 174 calories | 27 g carbohydrates | 7 g fat | 3 g protein |

| | |
|---|---|
| 5 to 6 (3- to 4-in.) beets | ½ cup balsamic vinegar |
| 2 TB. olive oil | 2 tsp. pure maple syrup (Grade B recommended) |
| ¼ tsp. sea salt | |
| ¼ tsp. freshly ground black pepper | 1 tsp. freshly grated orange zest |

1. Preheat oven to 325°F.

2. Wash beets and slice into quarters. Cut each quarter into ¼-inch slices.

3. Put beets on a baking sheet. Add olive oil, sea salt, and pepper and mix together completely. Spread beets out again on the baking sheet.

4. Roast for 45 minutes to an hour, checking often.

5. Mix balsamic vinegar and maple syrup together in a small pan over high heat. Cook until balsamic vinegar has reduced to a syruplike consistency. Remove from heat.

6. When beets are fully cooked, separate onto plates. Pour glaze over top and sprinkle with orange zest before serving.

**Variation:** You can use any root vegetable in place of the beets. Garnet yams, parsnips, and celery root are all excellent substitutions.

# Roasted Cauliflower with Tahini Sauce

Roasting cauliflower in a hot oven gives it a crisp texture on the outside, and toasty flavor on the inside. Perfect when paired with the tart tahini sauce.

| Yield: | Prep time: | Cook time: | Serving size: |
|---|---|---|---|
| 4 cups | 15 minutes | 30 minutes | 1 cup |

| Each serving has: | | | |
|---|---|---|---|
| 197 calories | 12 g carbohydrates | 15 g fat | 5 g protein |

2 TB. olive oil

2 tsp. ground cumin

1 head cauliflower, cored and cut into 1½-in. florets

Kosher salt

Freshly ground black pepper

½ cup tahini

3 cloves garlic, smashed into a paste

Juice of 1 lemon

½ cup water

1. Preheat oven to 500°F. Toss together olive oil, cumin, and cauliflower in a large bowl. Season to taste with kosher salt and pepper.

2. Transfer to a rimmed baking sheet; spread out evenly. Bake, rotating pan from top to bottom and front to back, until cauliflower is browned and tender, about 25 to 30 minutes.

3. Combine tahini, garlic, lemon juice, and water in a small bowl and season to taste with kosher salt. Serve cauliflower hot or at room temperature with tahini sauce.

**PALEO COMPASS**

You can find tahini (sesame seed butter) in Middle Eastern markets or at natural food grocers.

# Rosemary Green Beans

This simple and savory version is excellent as a fall or winter side dish.

| Yield: | Prep time: | Cook time: | Serving size: |
|---|---|---|---|
| 2 cups | 5 minutes | 20 minutes | ½ cup |

| Each serving has: | | | |
|---|---|---|---|
| 75 calories | 6 g carbohydrates | 6 g fat | 2 g protein |

1 lb. fresh green beans, trimmed

½ tsp. salt

2 green onions, sliced

2 tsp. fresh rosemary, chopped

1 tsp. olive oil

¼ cup chopped pecans, toasted (or almonds or other nut of your choice)

2 tsp. grated lemon rind

1. Sprinkle green beans evenly with ¼ teaspoon salt and place in a steamer basket over boiling water. Cover and steam 10 minutes or until crisp-tender.

2. Plunge green beans into ice water to stop cooking and drain.

3. Sauté green onions and rosemary in hot olive oil in a nonstick skillet over medium-high heat for 2 to 3 minutes or until softened.

4. Add green beans, pecans, lemon rind, and remaining ¼ teaspoon salt, stirring until thoroughly heated. Garnish and serve immediately.

# Sautéed Fennel and Carrots

This recipe comes close to making vegetables taste like candy.

| Yield: | Prep time: | Cook time: | Serving size: |
|---|---|---|---|
| 4 cups | 5 minutes | 25 minutes | 1 cup |

| Each serving has: | | | |
|---|---|---|---|
| 131 calories | 17 g carbohydrates | 7 g fat | 3 g protein |

| | |
|---|---|
| 2 fennel bulbs | Sea salt |
| 4 medium carrots | Freshly ground black pepper |
| 2 TB. coconut oil | |

1. Wash fennel bulbs and carrots and cut into ¼- to ½-inch-thick slices.

2. Heat coconut oil in a skillet over medium heat.

3. When the pan is hot, add fennel bulbs and carrots. Cook until tender, stirring occasionally.

4. Season to taste with sea salt and pepper and serve hot.

**PALEO COMPASS**

Save fennel fronds for a pretty eatable garnish, or add to your next salad or sautéed veggies. They are also great with baked salmon.

# Spicy Spaghetti Squash with Almonds

This recipe will have you cooking squash like a pro.

| Yield: | Prep time: | Cook time: | Serving size: |
|---|---|---|---|
| 4 cups | 20 minutes | 60 minutes | 1 cup |
| **Each serving has:** | | | |
| 124 calories | 6 g carbohydrates | 11 g fat | 3 g protein |

| | |
|---|---|
| 1 large spaghetti squash | ½ or 1 tsp. ground chipotle |
| ½ cup slivered almonds | ½ tsp. sea salt |
| 1 TB. coconut oil | ⅛ tsp. freshly grated nutmeg |

1. Preheat oven to 375°F.

2. Cut spaghetti squash in half lengthwise with a large knife or cleaver.

3. Place cut side down in a shallow baking dish. Add ¾ inch of water to the dish.

4. Bake for 45 minutes or so, until squash is soft to the touch.

5. Add slivered almonds to a small sauté pan over medium-low heat. Stir constantly until almonds turn golden brown. (Note: almonds will burn quickly if not stirred or if left unattended!) Set aside.

6. When squash is done cooking, remove from the oven and cool until it can be comfortably handled.

7. Turn the cut side up, and remove squash from rind with a fork. This should be done crosswise, so strands of squash fall out like spaghetti.

8. Toss spaghetti squash strands in coconut oil, ground chipotle, sea salt, and nutmeg, and top with toasted almonds. Serve warm or cold.

**Variation:** Spaghetti squash is an excellent alternative to traditional spaghetti. Cook the squash as indicated above, and top with tomato sauce, Mojo Verde (see the recipe later in this chapter), or additional sautéed vegetables for a satisfying alternative.

# Vegetable Kebabs

Ginger and garlic make these grilled kebabs a tasty summertime treat.

| Yield: | Prep time: | Cook time: | Serving size: |
|---|---|---|---|
| 8 to 10 kebabs | 15 minutes | 10 minutes | 4 kebabs |

| Each serving has: | | | |
|---|---|---|---|
| 408 calories | 37 g carbohydrates | 29 g fat | 8 g protein |

4 large cremini mushrooms, quartered

1 medium zucchini, sliced thick

½ head cauliflower, pulled apart into large florets

1 red bell pepper, cut into large pieces

1 medium white onion, cut into large pieces

1 (2-in.) piece fresh ginger root, peeled

2 cloves garlic

½ cup olive oil

½ tsp. cayenne

1 tsp. basil

1 tsp. oregano

10 wooden skewers

1. Place cremini mushrooms, zucchini, cauliflower, red bell pepper, and white onion in a large bowl.

2. Blend ginger root, garlic, olive oil, cayenne, basil, and oregano together in a blender or food processor and pour over vegetables in the bowl.

3. Cover and marinate overnight in the refrigerator.

4. Soak the wooden skewers in water overnight (or for at least 15 minutes before using) to prevent burning.

5. At mealtime, put vegetables onto the skewers.

6. Place kebabs on the grill for about 10 minutes until tender, turning frequently.

7. Remove vegetables from the skewers and serve immediately.

**PALEO COMPASS**

Don't skip the marinade time! While it may seem easy to toss the vegetables in the marinade and grill immediately, the flavor will certainly be lacking. Give the vegetables at least 4 hours to marinate, but overnight is better.

# Zucchini and Squash Sauté

The tomato sauce is a great addition to enhance the flavor of this dish.

| Yield: | Prep time: | Cook time: | Serving size: |
|---|---|---|---|
| 4 cups | 15 minutes | 20 minutes | 1 cup |
| **Each serving has:** | | | |
| 87 calories | 12 g carbohydrates | 4 g fat | 4 g protein |

1 TB. coconut oil

½ yellow onion, thinly sliced

2 cloves garlic, minced

2 (6- to 8-in.) zucchini, cut into 3×¼-in. matchsticks

2 (6- to 8-in.) yellow summer squash, cut into 3×¼-in. matchsticks

1 (6-oz.) can tomato sauce

1. In a large skillet, heat coconut oil over medium-high heat. When hot, add yellow onion and cook 3 to 4 minutes until onion is tender and translucent.

2. Add garlic, zucchini, and yellow summer squash, and cook until almost tender (5 to 6 minutes).

3. Stir in tomato sauce and cook until heated through. Serve warm.

**Variation:** For a more versatile accompaniment, eliminate the tomato sauce from this recipe to have a subtle side dish that pairs well with everything.

# Watermelon with Fresh Herbs

You may never eat plain watermelon again!

| Yield: | Prep time: | Serving size: | |
|---|---|---|---|
| 4 cups | 10 minutes | 1 cup | |
| **Each serving has:** | | | |
| 86 calories | 22 g carbohydrates | 1 g fat | 2 g protein |

¼ large watermelon                    ¼ cup fresh cilantro, chopped

1. Chop watermelon into 1-inch pieces, removing seeds, and put into a large bowl.

2. Add cilantro to watermelon and mix together. Serve chilled.

**Variation:** Use any fresh herbs you like (such as parsley, basil, mint, or oregano), or try a combination.

# Mojo Verde

This quick and easy sauce is excellent with grilled meats, or try it over cooked spaghetti squash.

| Yield: | Prep time: | Serving size: | |
|---|---|---|---|
| 1 cup | 10 minutes | ¼ cup | |
| **Each serving has:** | | | |
| 176 calories | 3 g carbohydrates | 18 g fat | 1 g protein |

2 cups fresh cilantro                    1 to 2 cloves garlic
¼ to ½ cup olive oil                     ½ tsp. sea salt

1. Blend cilantro, olive oil, garlic, and sea salt in a food processor until desired consistency is reached.

2. Store in an airtight container in the refrigerator until ready to use.

**Variation:** Don't like cilantro? Try using flat-leaf parsley or fresh basil instead.

# Mayonnaise

It's beneficial to make your own and control the quality of ingredients, and the fresh flavors and quality olive oil will really make the flavors stand out.

| Yield: | Prep time: | Serving size: | |
|---|---|---|---|
| 1½ cups | 15 minutes | 1½ tablespoons | |
| **Each serving has:** | | | |
| 106 calories | 0 g carbohydrates | 12 g fat | 0 g protein |

1 egg (safest if from pastured chickens)

½ tsp. lemon juice

½ cup olive oil

½ cup flaxseed oil

1. Combine egg and lemon juice in a blender.

2. Add 1 drop olive oil and continue to blend on high for 30 seconds.

3. Add 2 more drops olive oil and blend for 30 seconds.

4. Add 5 more drops olive oil and blend for 30 seconds.

5. Continue to slowly incorporate olive oil in small portions. The consistency of mayonnaise should begin to develop.

6. When olive oil is completely incorporated, slowly drizzle flaxseed oil into the blender and continue to blend.

7. Spoon into an airtight container and store in the refrigerator until ready to use.

**Variation:** Incorporate 1 clove garlic into step 1 and increase lemon juice to 1 tablespoon to make aioli.

# Simple Salad Dressing

Keep this simple dressing on hand to quickly add flavor to salads anytime.

| Yield: | Prep time: | Serving size: | |
|---|---|---|---|
| 16 tablespoons | 10 minutes | 2 tablespoons | |
| **Each serving has:** | | | |
| 254 calories | 4 g carbohydrates | 28 g fat | 0 g protein |

¼ cup balsamic vinegar

1 tsp. Dijon mustard

1 garlic clove, finely minced

1 tsp. raw honey

1 TB. lemon juice

1 cup olive oil

1 tsp. sea salt

½ tsp. freshly ground black pepper

1 TB. dried herbs of choice (basil, thyme, chives, rosemary, oregano, tarragon)

1. Whisk (or put in a blender) balsamic vinegar, Dijon mustard, minced garlic, raw honey, and lemon juice until blended.

2. Gradually add olive oil while whisking (or blending).

3. Add sea salt, pepper, and dried herbs.

4. Store in an airtight container in the refrigerator. Shake before using.

# Flavorful Fish and Seafood

## In This Chapter

- Hearty fish dishes
- The lighter side of fish
- A trio of savory shrimp dishes
- Enjoy the delicate flavor of fresh crab

Fish and seafood are an excellent departure from your everyday chicken and beef, and they have a lot of nutritional merits to boot. They're packed with protein, and many species contain an abundance of anti-inflammatory omega-3 fatty acids.

The following recipes, like the Chipotle Lime Salmon and the Green Lightning Shrimp, will help you expand your fish and seafood horizons. Note: when preparing fish, first rinse the fillet and pat dry before checking for bones.

# Almond Crusted Salmon

The nutty coating is an excellent match for the rich flavor of the salmon.

| Yield: | Prep time: | Cook time: | Serving size: |
|---|---|---|---|
| 1 lb. salmon fillet | 10 minutes | 15 minutes | ½ lb. salmon fillet |

| Each serving has: | | | |
|---|---|---|---|
| 431 calories | 7 g carbohydrates | 26 g fat | 44 g protein |

½ cup almond flour

½ tsp. ground coriander

½ tsp. ground cumin

1 lb. salmon fillet

Juice of 1 lemon

Sea salt

Freshly ground black pepper

½ tsp. coconut oil

2 sprigs fresh cilantro, chopped

1. Preheat the oven to 500°F.

2. Combine almond meal, coriander, and cumin in a small bowl.

3. Sprinkle salmon fillets with lemon juice and season to taste with sea salt and pepper.

4. Coat each fillet with almond meal mixture.

5. Place fish skin side down on a broiler pan, greased lightly with coconut oil.

6. Bake for 15 minutes, or until salmon flakes easily with a fork.

7. Top with cilantro before serving.

# Chipotle Lime Salmon

This recipe will satisfy your craving for something a little bit spicy. Adjust the amount of chipotle as desired.

| Yield: | Prep time: | Cook time: | Serving size: |
| --- | --- | --- | --- |
| 1 lb. salmon fillet | 5 minutes | 15 minutes | ½ lb. salmon fillet |
| **Each serving has:** | | | |
| 519 calories | 8 g carbohydrates | 21 g fat | 49 g protein |

1 lb. salmon fillet

1 to 2 TB. olive oil

2 limes, cut in half

1 tsp. sea salt (optional)

1 tsp. ground chipotle

1. Preheat oven to 500°F.

2. Rinse salmon, pat dry, and place on a metal baking sheet.

3. Rub each fillet with olive oil, and squeeze the juice from one-half lime onto each fillet.

4. Sprinkle fillet with sea salt (if using) and chipotle, then place a half-lime on top of each fillet.

5. Turn down oven temperature to 275°F and immediately place salmon in oven. Cook for 8 to 12 minutes, or until salmon is cooked to the desired temperature.

6. When salmon flakes easily with a fork, remove from oven and serve hot.

**PALEO COMPASS**

Try this recipe on the grill for an easy summertime meal.

# Fish and Vegetable Curry

The coconut milk helps tame the spicy curry in this easy dish.

| Yield: | Prep time: | Cook time: | Serving size: |
|---|---|---|---|
| 4 cups | 15 minutes | 15 minutes | 2 cups |

| Each serving has: | | | |
|---|---|---|---|
| 380 calories | 30 g carbohydrates | 14 g fat | 45 g protein |

1 (13.6-oz.) can unsweetened coconut milk

2 TB. red curry paste

2 medium carrots, cut into thin matchsticks

½ small red cabbage, thinly sliced

1 lb. white fish fillets, cut crosswise into 1-in. slices

¼ cup fresh cilantro, chopped

1. Put coconut milk and red curry paste in a large sauté pan over medium heat. Cook for 3 minutes, stirring until combined.

2. Add carrots and red cabbage to pan. Cover and simmer for 4 to 5 minutes.

3. Add white fish fillets and simmer an additional 4 to 5 minutes, or until fish is fully cooked.

4. Serve with fresh cilantro.

# Salmon Cakes with Mango and Cilantro Salsa

This dish is sweet and salty, with a crisp salad on the side.

| Yield: | Prep time: | Cook time: | Serving size: |
|---|---|---|---|
| 8 (3-in.) salmon cakes with salsa | 15 minutes | 10 minutes | 4 (3-in.) salmon cakes with salsa |

| Each serving has: | | | |
|---|---|---|---|
| 729 calories | 28 g carbohydrates | 38 g fat | 61 g protein |

| | |
|---|---|
| 1 lb. salmon fillet, skinless, with bones removed | 1 jalapeño pepper, minced |
| 2 eggs | 1 TB. coconut oil |
| 2 TB. coconut flour | 1 large ripe mango, diced |
| ½ tsp. plus dash sea salt | ½ cup red onion, minced |
| ¼ tsp. white pepper | 4 TB. chopped cilantro |
| | 1 TB. olive oil |

1. Check salmon carefully to be sure all bones have been removed. Chop into a fine dice and set aside.

2. Beat eggs in a large bowl. Mix in coconut flour, ½ teaspoon sea salt, and white pepper.

3. Add jalapeño pepper to the egg mixture. Add salmon and combine completely.

4. Warm a skillet over medium-high heat, and add coconut oil when pan is hot.

5. Test the pan to be sure it is hot by dropping a tiny portion of salmon mixture in the pan—it should sizzle immediately.

6. Add salmon mixture to coconut oil in small 3-inch cakes and fry until they are golden brown on the outside, and cooked pink on the inside (1 or 2 minutes on each side). Let the cakes rest on paper towels when taken out of the pan to absorb any extra coconut oil.

7. Meanwhile, prepare salsa by combining mango, red onion, and cilantro in a bowl. Drizzle with olive oil and add remaining dash sea salt. Serve on top of salmon cakes.

**Variation:** Replace the salmon with 1 pound cooked crab for an excellent alternative.

# Salmon with Coconut Cream Sauce

This rich and delicious entrée will even impress your non-Paleo friends.

| Yield: | Prep time: | Cook time: | Serving size: |
|---|---|---|---|
| 1¾ lb. salmon fillet | 10 minutes | 30 minutes | 8 oz. fish fillet |
| **Each serving has:** | | | |
| 539 calories | 10 g carbohydrates | 37 g fat | 44 g protein |

1¾ lb. salmon fillet

½ tsp. sea salt (optional)

¼ tsp. freshly ground black pepper

1 TB. coconut oil

6 cloves garlic, minced

2 large shallots, diced

Zest and juice of 2 lemons

1 (13.6-oz.) can coconut milk

3 TB. fresh basil, chopped

1. Preheat oven to 350°F.

2. Place salmon in a shallow baking dish and sprinkle both sides with sea salt (if using) and pepper.

3. Heat a large sauté pan over medium heat. When pan is hot, add coconut oil, garlic, and shallots. Sauté until garlic and shallots soften, about 3 to 5 minutes.

4. Add lemon zest, lemon juice, and coconut milk, and bring liquid to a low boil.

5. Reduce heat and add basil.

6. Pour mixture over salmon and bake uncovered for about 10 to 20 minutes, or until salmon has reached desired temperature.

7. When salmon flakes with a fork, remove from heat and serve hot.

# Baked Sea Bass with Capers and Lemon

This mouthwatering recipe enhances the subtle flavors of the sea bass.

| Yield: | Prep time: | Cook time: | Serving size: |
| --- | --- | --- | --- |
| 1 lb. sea bass fillet | 5 minutes | 15 minutes | 8 oz. sea bass fillet |
| **Each serving has:** | | | |
| 243 calories | 12 g carbohydrates | 5 g fat | 41 g protein |

| | |
| --- | --- |
| 1 lb. sea bass fillet | 2 TB. capers, rinsed |
| ½ tsp. coconut oil | 2 sprigs fresh dill |
| ½ tsp. sea salt (optional) | 1 lemon, thinly sliced |
| Freshly ground black pepper | |

1. Preheat oven to 350°F.

2. Lightly grease broiler pan with coconut oil and place sea bass fillets on pan.

3. Sprinkle with sea salt (if using) and pepper. Top with capers and dill. Cover with lemon slices.

4. Bake for 10 to 15 minutes, until fish flakes easily with a fork. Serve hot.

**Variation:** Replace the sea bass with cod, tilapia, halibut, or any other firm white fish.

# Cod with Arugula Tapenade and Celeriac Fries

This recipe looks complicated, but it's actually incredibly easy to make. Try it for a dinner party to show off your cooking skills.

| Yield: | Prep time: | Cook time: | Serving size: |
|---|---|---|---|
| 1 lb. fish and 2 cups fries | 15 minutes | 20 minutes | ½ lb. fish and 1 cup fries |

| Each serving has: | | | |
|---|---|---|---|
| 286 calories | 24 g carbohydrates | 11 g fat | 26 g protein |

1 head celeriac, or celery root, peeled and cut into ¼-in. strips

2 tsp. olive oil

Sea salt (optional)

Freshly ground black pepper (optional)

2 cod fillets

Juice of 1 lemon

1 small bunch (about ¼ lb.) arugula

½ cup green or black olives, pitted

2 TB. capers, rinsed

1 or 2 cloves garlic, roughly chopped

1. Preheat oven to 450°F.

2. Cut celeriac into ¼-inch strips (like French fries) and place in an oven-proof dish. Drizzle with olive oil and season to taste with sea salt (if using) and pepper (if using).

3. Bake fries for approximately 10 minutes.

4. Place cod fillets in another oven-proof dish and season to taste with sea salt (if using), pepper (if using), and lemon juice.

5. After celeriac has baked for 10 minutes, decrease the temperature to 400°F and bake cod together with fries for another 8 to 10 minutes.

6. While cod bakes, combine arugula, green olives, capers, and garlic in a food processor and chop until it resembles a tapenade.

7. Serve tapenade on top of cod, with celeriac fries on the side.

# Louisiana Fillets

Just as scrumptious as what's served in the deep South, but so much healthier for you.

| Yield: | Prep time: | Cook time: | Serving size: |
|---|---|---|---|
| 1 lb. fillet | 10 minutes | 25 minutes | ½ fillet |

| Each serving has: | | | |
|---|---|---|---|
| 275 calories | 2 g carbohydrates | 16 g fat | 31 g protein |

| | |
|---|---|
| 2 TB. coconut oil | ⅛ tsp. crushed red pepper |
| Juice of 1 lemon | ⅛ tsp. garlic powder |
| 1 lb. firm white fish fillet (sole, trout, snapper, or catfish) | Sea salt (optional) |
| ½ tsp. lemon pepper | Freshly ground black pepper (optional) |

1. Preheat oven to 350°F.

2. In a medium oven-proof skillet, heat coconut oil and lemon juice over medium-high heat.

3. Coat both sides of white fish fillets with oil mixture and lay fish side by side in the pan, overlapping slightly if necessary.

4. Mix lemon pepper, red pepper, and garlic powder together and sprinkle over fillets.

5. Bake for 20 to 25 minutes, depending on size of fillets and type of fish. (Catfish bakes the longest.)

6. The pan may blacken, but that's fine; the liquid will keep fish moist.

7. Season to taste with sea salt (if using) and pepper (if using).

8. When fish flakes easily with a fork, remove from heat and serve hot.

**Variation:** For a truly southern treat, pan-fry the fish in ¼ cup bacon drippings.

# Macadamia-Encrusted Halibut

This pleasing dish is eye-catching when served with colorful orange slices.

| Yield: | Prep time: | Cook time: | Serving size: |
|---|---|---|---|
| 1 lb. halibut | 20 minutes | 15 minutes | ½ lb. halibut |

| Each serving has: | | | |
|---|---|---|---|
| 693 calories | 17 g carbohydrates | 49 g fat | 52 g protein |

¾ cup Macadamia nuts

1 tsp. olive oil

1 egg

2 tsp. unsweetened almond or coconut milk

1 TB. fresh parsley, chopped

¼ tsp. sea salt (optional)

¼ tsp. freshly ground black pepper

Zest of ½ orange

1 lb. fresh halibut fillet

1 orange, sliced

1. Preheat oven to 350°F.

2. Toast Macadamia nuts in a small skillet over medium-low heat until slightly golden. Note: stir constantly, as nuts will burn quickly if unattended. Set aside and allow nuts to cool completely before chopping. Chop when cool.

3. Lightly grease a shallow baking dish with olive oil.

4. In a medium bowl, beat egg with almond milk and set aside.

5. Add parsley, sea salt (if using), pepper, and orange zest to a shallow bowl with nuts.

6. Dip each halibut fillet in egg mixture, and coat on both sides, then press halibut in nut mixture. Be sure each fillet is fully coated with mixture.

7. Place fillets in the shallow baking pan, and bake for 15 minutes (or until fish flakes apart with a fork).

8. Serve with orange slices.

# Red Snapper Azteca

Red snapper fillets are heavenly with the spicy components of this meal.

| Yield: | Prep time: | Cook time: | Serving size: |
|---|---|---|---|
| 1 lb. fish fillet | 15 minutes | 30 minutes | ½ lb. fish fillet |
| **Each serving has:** | | | |
| 341 calories | 11 g carbohydrates | 4 g fat | 64 g protein |

| | |
|---|---|
| 1 lb. red snapper fillet | 1 plum tomato, coarsely chopped |
| Juice of 1 lime | 1 small Anaheim pepper, chopped |
| Juice of ½ lemon | ½ red bell pepper, chopped |
| 1 tsp. chili powder | Handful fresh cilantro, chopped |
| 4 green onions, sliced in ½-in. sections | |

1. Place red snapper in a shallow baking dish.

2. Combine lime juice, lemon juice, and chili powder in small bowl and drizzle over snapper.

3. Preheat oven to 350°F.

4. Marinate fish for 10 minutes, turning a few times.

5. Sprinkle chopped green onions, tomato, Anaheim pepper, and red bell pepper over snapper.

6. Cover and bake for 20 to 30 minutes or just until snapper flakes in center.

7. Let stand, covered, 4 minutes.

8. Garnish with fresh cilantro before serving.

# Steamed Flounder Rolls

This delicious meal is an easy way to incorporate additional root vegetables into your diet.

| Yield: | Prep time: | Cook time: | Serving size: |
|---|---|---|---|
| 1 lb. fillet | 15 minutes | 15 minutes | ½ lb. fillet |

| Each serving has: | | | |
|---|---|---|---|
| 459 calories | 38 g carbohydrates | 18 g fat | 39 g protein |

1 lb. flounder fillet

Sea salt

Freshly ground black pepper

2 TB. coconut oil

2 medium carrots, sliced into ¼×2-in. matchsticks

2 small parsnips, sliced into ¼×2-in. matchsticks

2 leeks (white and light green sections only), rinsed thoroughly and sliced

1 to 1½ cups vegetable broth

1 tsp. thyme

1. Cut fish fillets in half lengthwise.

2. Season each piece with sea salt and pepper, and roll into small rolls.

3. Heat a large sauté pan over medium-high heat. Add coconut oil to pan when hot.

4. Add carrots, parsnips, and leeks to the pan and sauté for about 5 minutes.

5. Reduce heat to low, and add vegetable broth and thyme.

6. Place fish rolls on top of vegetables and cover.

7. Steam for 8 to 10 minutes or until fish is tender. Note: do not remove lid unless necessary to check for doneness.

# Coconut Shrimp

A delectable combination of garlic, coconut, and ginger makes this dish irresistible.

| Yield: | Prep time: | Cook time: | Serving size: |
|---|---|---|---|
| 30 to 40 shrimp | 10 minutes | 20 minutes | 15 to 20 shrimp |

| Each serving has: | | | |
|---|---|---|---|
| 371 calories | 10 g carbohydrates | 18 g fat | 43 g protein |

| | |
|---|---|
| 1 lb. raw shrimp or prawns (31 to 40 count), in shell | 1 tsp. ginger root, peeled and minced |
| 1 (13.6-oz.) can coconut milk | ¼ tsp. sea salt |
| 1 or 2 cloves garlic, minced | ¼ tsp. freshly ground black pepper |

1. Wash shrimp, but do not shell them.

2. Place shrimp into a medium saucepan with coconut milk, garlic, ginger root, sea salt, and pepper.

3. Bring to a boil, stirring frequently.

4. Reduce heat and simmer uncovered until shrimp are pink and firm. Stir frequently. Serve.

# Green Lightning Shrimp

The summer flavors in this dish are sure to make it a favorite.

| Yield: | Prep time: | Cook time: | Serving size: |
|---|---|---|---|
| 21 to 24 shrimp | 40 minutes | 10 minutes | 10 to 12 shrimp |
| **Each serving has:** | | | |
| 497 calories | 8 g carbohydrates | 38 g fat | 29 g protein |

1 lb. jumbo shrimp (21 to 25 count), peeled and deveined

10 metal or bamboo skewers (2 for each shrimp)

1 bunch (about 1 cup) cilantro, rinsed and coarsely chopped

3 cloves garlic, chopped

4 jalapeño peppers, seeded and coarsely chopped (for hotter shrimp, leave the seeds in)

6 green onions, chopped

1 tsp. sea salt

1 tsp. freshly ground black pepper

1 tsp. ground cumin

½ cup olive oil

Juice of 2 limes plus 2 additional limes cut into wedges

1. Thread shrimp onto skewers, using two skewers for each kebab. Arrange the kebabs in a shallow glass or ceramic dish.

2. Set aside 3 tablespoons chopped cilantro and 2 garlic cloves for garlic-cilantro sauce. Place remaining cilantro, jalapeño peppers, green onions, remaining 1 clove garlic, sea salt, black pepper, and cumin in a food processor and finely chop. With the machine running, add ¼ cup olive oil and lime juice through the feed tube and purée. Pour over shrimp and let marinate in the refrigerator, covered, for 30 minutes.

3. Shortly before mealtime, heat remaining ¼ cup olive oil in a small saucepan over medium heat. When pan is hot, add reserved garlic and cilantro and cook until garlic is golden and fragrant, about 2 minutes. Keep garlic-cilantro sauce warm until ready to use.

4. Prepare the grill.

5. When ready to cook, drain and discard marinade from kebabs. Place shrimp kebabs on the hot grill and baste with garlic-cilantro sauce. Continue to baste and grill until just cooked through, 1 to 3 minutes per side, until shrimp are pinkish white and firm.

6. Pour any remaining garlic-cilantro sauce over top and serve with fresh lime wedges.

# Grilled Shrimp and Veggies on a Stick

This fun recipe is an excellent addition to an outdoor party.

| Yield: | Prep time: | Cook time: | Serving size: |
|---|---|---|---|
| 6 skewers | 30 minutes | 10 minutes | 3 skewers |
| **Each serving has:** | | | |
| 460 calories | 26 g carbohydrates | 24 g fat | 38 g protein |

6 wooden skewers

¾ lb. shrimp, peeled and deveined

Juice of 1 lime

Freshly ground black pepper

1 medium zucchini, sliced into 1-in. pieces

1 medium yellow summer squash, sliced into 1-in. pieces

1 red bell pepper, sliced into 2-in. pieces

1 green bell pepper, sliced into 2-in. pieces

1 red onion, cut into eighths

4 cloves garlic, minced

3 TB. olive oil

1. Soak wooden skewers in water for at least 15 minutes to prevent burning.

2. Place shrimp in a medium bowl. Add lime juice and season with black pepper. Set aside for 5 minutes.

3. Prepare the grill.

4. Add zucchini, yellow summer squash, red bell pepper, green bell pepper, red onion, and garlic to shrimp, and add olive oil. Toss.

5. Alternately thread vegetables and shrimp onto the skewers.

6. Grill until fully cooked, about 3 to 5 minutes per side, and serve warm.

# Dill and Lime Crab

The delicately sweet flavor of fresh Dungeness crab is unbeatable.

| Yield: | Prep time: | Cook time: | Serving size: |
|---|---|---|---|
| 2 (1-lb.) crabs | 20 minutes | 15 minutes | 1 crab |

| Each serving has: | | | |
|---|---|---|---|
| 158 calories | 7 g carbohydrates | 2 g fat | 29 g protein |

2 large (¾- to 1-lb.) Dungeness crabs

Juice of 1 lime plus 1 additional lime

1 tsp. paprika

2 tsp. fresh dill, chopped

1. Heat a stockpot full of water over high heat until boiling.

2. Once boiling, carefully drop in Dungeness crabs, using tongs.

3. Cover partially, and cook for 7 to 8 minutes.

4. Carefully remove crabs from water, and run under cold water until cool enough to handle.

5. Once cool, crack and clean shells, and remove meat.

6. Drizzle meat with lime juice and sprinkle with paprika and dill.

7. Serve with lime wedges.

**PALEO COMPASS**

Dungeness crab season begins in November or December along the West Coast, and continues until June.

# Tasty Beef, Bison, Lamb, and Pork

## In This Chapter

- Meaty meals in 30 minutes or less
- Family favorites in under an hour
- Flavorful fare with a Paleo twist
- Chill-chasing, one-pot meals

Meat is full of protein, iron, zinc, and the highly valued B vitamins. Not many foods offer as much vitamin B, iron, and alpha lipoic acid (a powerful antioxidant) as red meat. Sometimes it's difficult to make your meat taste like more than just meat, though. We all want to make pork loin or steak worthy of a 5-star restaurant, and now you can! The following recipes for beef, bison, lamb, and pork are full of new and exciting, complex flavors.

We'll start off with quick meals like the Bun-Less Burgers and Lime-Cilantro Pork Wraps that take 30 minutes or less to prepare. Then we'll progress to dishes that take more time, up to 7 hours, like the Slow Cooker Pork Loin.

# Bun-Less Burgers

This simple standby is quick, delicious, and may easily become a weekly favorite. (Note: nutritional information is based on 85 percent lean ground beef.)

| Yield: | Prep time: | Cooking time: | Serving size: |
|---|---|---|---|
| 4 burgers | 5 minutes | 20 minutes | 1 burger |
| **Each serving has:** | | | |
| 200 calories | 0 g carbohydrates | 11 g fat | 23 g protein |

1 lb. lean ground beef or turkey

½ tsp. sea salt

¼ tsp. freshly ground black pepper

1 tsp. coconut oil

1. Mix beef, sea salt, and pepper together with a fork. Form into 4 patties.

2. Heat a skillet over medium-high heat and add coconut oil when hot.

3. Cook burgers until desired temperature is reached and serve hot.

# Coconut Lamb with Cauliflower "Rice"

The coconut milk and fresh ginger in this dinner help to balance the pungent flavor of the lamb.

| Yield: | Prep time: | Cook time: | Serving size: |
|---|---|---|---|
| 1 lb. lamb and 6 cups vegetables | 15 minutes | 15 minutes | 4 oz. lamb and 1½ cups vegetables |
| **Each serving has:** | | | |
| 454 calories | 26 g carbohydrates | 32 g fat | 33 g protein |

3 TB. coconut oil

½ sweet yellow onion, diced

1 large carrot, cut in ¼-in. slices

1 lb. lamb (tenderloin or steak), cubed

4 medium tomatoes, diced

2 (13.6-oz.) cans coconut milk

2 medium zucchini, cut in ¼-in. slices

1 head cauliflower

½ tsp. ground ginger

½ tsp. sea salt

¼ tsp. freshly ground black pepper

3 TB. fresh cilantro, chopped

1. Over medium-high heat, add 1 tablespoon coconut oil to a large pan.

2. When the pan is hot, add yellow onions and carrots (they should sizzle slightly). Cook until onions are slightly translucent.

3. Add lamb, tomatoes, and coconut milk. Simmer uncovered for 20 to 30 minutes or until lamb is fully cooked and tender.

4. Add zucchini to lamb mixture and continue to simmer for 5 to 10 more minutes.

5. Rough-chop cauliflower and place in a large skillet with remaining 2 tablespoons coconut oil. Cook over medium-high heat until slightly softened.

6. Place cauliflower with ginger into a food processor and pulse until it has a grainy ricelike consistency. Season with sea salt and pepper.

7. Season lamb mixture with additional sea salt and pepper. Add cilantro and serve over cauliflower rice.

**Variation:** When making the cauliflower rice, use any additional seasonings desired—garlic powder, coconut aminos, curry, or chili powder.

# Lime-Cilantro Pork Wraps

Fresh and spicy! This recipe makes a great, quick weeknight meal.

| Yield: | Prep time: | Cook time: | Serving size: |
|---|---|---|---|
| 8 wraps | 15 minutes | 15 minutes | 2 wraps |

| Each serving has: | | | |
|---|---|---|---|
| 176 calories | 13 g carbohydrates | 5 g fat | 28 g protein |

1 lb. pork tenderloin, trimmed and cut into ¼- to ½-in. strips

¼ tsp. sea salt

⅛ tsp. freshly ground black pepper

2 tsp. coconut oil

1 red onion, diced

1 small jalapeño pepper, minced

½ cup chicken broth

1 medium tomato, diced

3 TB. lime juice

3 TB. cilantro, chopped

1 head butter lettuce

1. Season pork strips with sea salt and pepper.

2. Heat a large nonstick skillet over medium-high heat. When hot, add coconut oil to pan.

3. Sauté pork until lightly browned, about 4 minutes. Remove pork from pan and place in a bowl.

4. Add red onion and jalapeño pepper to hot pan, and sauté until tender.

5. Add chicken broth and tomato, and reduce heat to low. Simmer 2 minutes more, scraping pan sides and bottom to loosen any browned bits.

6. Return pork and juices to the pan. Stir in lime juice and simmer until pork is fully cooked.

7. Top with fresh cilantro and wrap in butter lettuce leaves to serve.

**Variation:** For a heartier version, substitute pork tenderloin with 1 pound sirloin beef steak, and use ½ cup beef broth instead of chicken broth. Season sirloin as indicated in recipe and then broil just until medium rare. Thinly slice beef across the grain and toss in with vegetables at the end.

# Pepper Steak

Enjoy the succulent flavor of a great steak with this easy recipe.

| Yield:<br>1 lb. steak and 4 cups vegetables | Prep time:<br>15 minutes | Cook time:<br>15 minutes | Serving size:<br>4 oz. steak and<br>1 cup vegetables |
| --- | --- | --- | --- |
| Each serving has:<br>420 calories | 13 g carbohydrates | 24 g fat | 39 g protein |

1 lb. beef round steak (about ½ in. thick)

2 TB. coconut or olive oil

1 medium yellow onion, sliced

1 medium green pepper, sliced

¼ cup water

¼ tsp. garlic salt

Freshly ground black pepper

4 large carrots, shredded

1. Cut steak into ¼- to ½-in. slices.

2. Add coconut oil to a large skillet over medium-high heat.

3. Brown meat and yellow onions in hot oil until onions turn slightly translucent.

4. Stir in green pepper, water, and garlic salt. Cook another 5 minutes, stirring constantly.

5. Season to taste with black pepper and serve on bed of shredded carrots.

# Sausage Stuffed Tomatoes

This recipe is best in late summer, when tomatoes are especially flavorful.

| Yield: | Prep time: | Cook time: | Serving size: |
|---|---|---|---|
| 6 stuffed tomatoes | 10 minutes | 20 minutes | 1½ stuffed tomatoes |

| Each serving has: | | | |
|---|---|---|---|
| 367 calories | 16 g carbohydrates | 27 g fat | 20 g protein |

1 medium yellow onion, chopped

1 lb. ground sausage, nitrite/nitrate free

6 white button mushrooms, sliced

6 large, very firm tomatoes

Fresh cilantro

1. Preheat oven to 350°F.

2. Over medium-high heat, brown yellow onions, sausage, and mushrooms together in a skillet.

3. While the mixture is cooking, cut tops off tomatoes. Spoon out tomato pulp and add to the skillet.

4. Once yellow onions, sausage, and mushrooms are cooked, drain fat and residual moisture from pan.

5. Spoon mixture into tomato cups.

6. Bake for 10 to 15 minutes.

7. Sprinkle with fresh cilantro before serving.

**Variation:** Use poblano or ancho peppers instead of large tomatoes. Simply cut off the top of the pepper and remove the seeds. Add 1 large tomato, diced, to onions and mushrooms and follow the recipe. Spoon the mixture into each pepper and bake for 25 minutes.

# Taco Salad

This taco salad is a great way to incorporate a variety of vegetables into one meal.

| Yield: | Prep time: | Cook time: | Serving size: |
|---|---|---|---|
| 8 cups | 10 minutes | 20 minutes | 2 cups |

| Each serving has: | | | |
|---|---|---|---|
| 329 calories | 15 g carbohydrates | 19 g fat | 26 g protein |

| | |
|---|---|
| 1 lb. lean ground beef or turkey | ¾ cup water |
| ½ yellow onion, diced | 3 romaine lettuce hearts |
| 2 TB. chili powder | 1 avocado, sliced |
| 1 tsp. garlic salt | 1 can black olives, sliced |
| 1 tsp. cumin | 1 medium tomato, diced |
| ½ tsp. oregano | Fresh cilantro |
| ½ tsp. sea salt | 1 (8-oz.) jar salsa |

1. Heat skillet over medium-high heat. Add beef and yellow onion to pan. Cook for about 10 minutes, or until browned.

2. Add chili powder, garlic salt, cumin, oregano, sea salt, and water, and let simmer for 5 minutes more.

3. Wash romaine lettuce and tear onto two plates (save some for leftovers).

4. Top romaine lettuce with meat and add sliced avocado, black olives, tomatoes, cilantro, and salsa before serving.

**Variation:** Use 1 pound of boneless, skinless chicken breasts in place of ground beef or turkey.

# Zucchini and Ground Beef

Zucchini never tasted so good! This meal is easy and inexpensive to prepare.

| Yield:<br>6 cups | Prep time:<br>15 minutes | Cook time:<br>15 minutes | Serving size:<br>1½ cups |
| --- | --- | --- | --- |
| **Each serving has:**<br>271 calories | 9 g carbohydrates | 15 g fat | 25 g protein |

1 TB. coconut oil

½ yellow onion, diced

1 lb. lean ground beef

1 or 2 cloves garlic, minced

2 TB. dried oregano

2 medium (6- to 8-in.) zucchini, diced

2 medium tomatoes, diced

1. Heat a large skillet over medium-high heat. Add coconut oil when hot.

2. Add yellow onions to the skillet and sauté until slightly translucent, about 5 minutes.

3. Add ground beef into pan, along with garlic and oregano. Cook 5 minutes, stirring occasionally.

4. Add zucchini and tomatoes and cook until tender. Serve hot.

# Easy Pork Loin Chops

Rich spices bring out the best in this quick pork chop recipe.

| Yield: | Prep time: | Cook time: | Serving size: |
|---|---|---|---|
| 4 pork chops | 10 minutes | 40 minutes | 1 pork chop |

| Each serving has: | | | |
|---|---|---|---|
| 234 calories | 4 g carbohydrates | 8 g fat | 34 g protein |

| | |
|---|---|
| ½ tsp. sea salt | ¼ tsp. dried thyme |
| ¼ tsp. freshly ground black pepper | 4 (4-oz.) boneless pork loin chops |
| ¼ tsp. paprika | 1 TB. coconut oil |
| ¼ tsp. dried sage | 1 yellow onion, sliced thin |

1. Preheat oven to 425°F.

2. In a small bowl, mix together sea salt, pepper, paprika, sage, and thyme.

3. Sprinkle both sides of each pork chop with seasoning mixture.

4. Add coconut oil to a skillet over high heat.

5. When hot, add pork chops and brown both sides of each chop.

6. Place browned chops on a large piece of heavy foil and layer with sliced yellow onions.

7. Close the foil into a tight pouch and place on a baking sheet.

8. Bake for 30 minutes, or until pork reaches desired temperature. Serve hot.

**PALEO COMPASS**

Undercooking any type of meat can be dangerous, and pork is no exception. With current USDA regulations and stricter inspection standards, the risks are lower than they used to be. Because of this, in 2011 the USDA lowered its recommended cooking temperature of pork to 145°F from the longtime standard of 160°F.

# Gingery Broccoli and Beef

This meal is easy to make in large quantities for balanced meals on the go during busy weeks.

| Yield: | Prep time: | Cook time: | Serving size: |
|---|---|---|---|
| 8 cups | 20 minutes | 25 minutes | 2 cups |

| Each serving has: | | | |
|---|---|---|---|
| 325 calories | 11 g carbohydrates | 16 g fat | 34 g protein |

2 TB. coconut oil

2 cloves garlic, minced

1 lb. petite sirloin steak, cut into very thin strips

¼ tsp. sea salt

2 TB. lemon juice

1 TB. flaxseeds, ground

2 tsp. fresh ginger root, grated

2 tsp. freshly ground black pepper

½ tsp. red pepper flakes

½ cup chicken broth, plus another ¼ cup (optional)

2 cups broccoli, cut into flowerets

2 cups carrots, thinly sliced

1 green onion, thinly sliced

1. Heat 1 tablespoon coconut oil and garlic in a large skillet over medium-high heat.

2. Add sliced sirloin and sea salt, and brown. Remove sirloin from pan to a side dish, and pour off excess juice left in pan.

3. In a small bowl, mix lemon juice, ground flaxseeds, grated ginger root, black pepper, and red pepper flakes with ½ cup chicken broth (plus additional ¼ cup, if using).

4. Heat the pan again over medium heat. Add remaining 1 tablespoon coconut oil when the pan is hot.

5. Add broccoli and carrots to pan. Pour liquid ingredients on top and toss to coat.

6. Cook over medium heat until broccoli is tender.

7. Return beef to the pan and add green onions. Add remaining ¼ cup chicken broth (if using).

8. Coat sirloin with sauce and let simmer for a few minutes until sirloin is warmed through. Serve hot.

# Grilled Flank Steak with Pineapple Salsa

This showstopper satisfies a craving for something sweet and spicy.

| Yield: | Prep time: | Cook time: | Serving size: |
|---|---|---|---|
| 1 lb. steak and 2 cups salsa | 20 minutes | 25 minutes | 4 oz. steak and 1 cup salsa |

| Each serving has: | | | |
|---|---|---|---|
| 255 calories | 10 g carbohydrates | 13 g fat | 25 g protein |

| | |
|---|---|
| 1 TB. olive oil | 1 large red bell pepper, diced |
| 1 tsp. chipotle powder | ½ red onion, diced |
| 1 lb. beef flank steak | ¼ cup cilantro, chopped |
| 4 slices fresh pineapple, cut into rings (canned pineapple in juice may be used) | Juice of 1 lime |

1. Prepare the grill or preheat the broiler to high.

2. Mix olive oil and chipotle powder together in a small bowl.

3. Brush onto both sides of beef flank steak.

4. Grill steak for around 5 minutes on one side, and 3 more minutes on the other. Or broil 3 minutes on one side and then 2 minutes on the other.

5. Move steak to a plate, cover, and let rest for 10 minutes.

6. Grill pineapple rings for 2 to 3 minutes per side, or broil for 45 seconds to 1 minute per side.

7. Cut pineapple rings into small chunks and place in a medium bowl.

8. Add red bell pepper, red onion, cilantro, and lime juice and mix together.

9. Slice steak thinly, and serve with pineapple salsa.

# Paleo Pizza

The soft crust on this pizza has a great texture!

| Yield: | Prep time: | Cook time: | Serving size: |
|---|---|---|---|
| 1 (12-in.) pizza | 15 minutes | 45 minutes | ¼ pizza |

| **Each serving has:** | | | |
|---|---|---|---|
| 459 calories | 38 g carbohydrates | 18 g fat | 39 g protein |

1 cup almond flour

3 TB. almond butter

2 eggs, beaten

½ tsp. sea salt

3 tsp. olive oil

½ cup yellow onion, diced

4 white button mushrooms, sliced

1 large Italian sausage, cut in ½-in. slices

2 cloves garlic, minced

1 red bell pepper, diced

½ cup marinara or tomato sauce, with no sugar added

½ tsp. dried oregano

½ tsp. fennel seed

½ cup cherry or grape tomatoes, sliced in half

1. Preheat oven to 350°F.

2. Mix almond flour, almond butter, eggs, and sea salt in a small bowl.

3. Coat a baking sheet with 2 teaspoons olive oil, then spread flour mixture over oil, making a ¼-inch-thick crust. Bake for 10 minutes.

4. While the crust is baking, add remaining 1 teaspoon olive oil, yellow onions, mushrooms, and sliced Italian sausage to a large skillet over medium-high heat and cook until Italian sausage is browned and onions are slightly translucent. Remove from the skillet and set aside.

5. Add garlic and red bell pepper to the skillet. Sauté vegetables for a few minutes, or until slightly tender. Note: do not cook vegetables entirely in the skillet or they will be too soft when cooked on the pizza.

6. Remove crust from the oven and cover with marinara sauce. Add Italian sausage and sautéed vegetables. Sprinkle with oregano and fennel seed, then bake for 20 to 30 minutes.

7. Remove from oven when fully cooked and top is golden brown. Top with sliced cherry tomatoes.

8. Carefully lift pizza off the baking sheet as the dough will still be soft. Cut into slices and serve.

# Pork Loin with Peppers, Mushrooms, and Onions

Caraway seeds add a subtle flavor to the pork in this meal that is unique and delicious.

| Yield: | Prep time: | Cook time: | Serving size: |
|---|---|---|---|
| 1 lb. pork and 2 cups vegetables | 15 minutes | 25 minutes | 4 oz. pork and 1 cup vegetables |

| Each serving has: | | | |
|---|---|---|---|
| 231 calories | 13 g carbohydrates | 6 g fat | 29 g protein |

| | |
|---|---|
| 1 lb. pork loin | 2 to 3 porcini mushrooms, sliced |
| 1 TB. caraway seeds | 2 red bell peppers, sliced |
| ½ tsp. sea salt | 4 cloves garlic, minced |
| ¼ tsp. freshly ground black pepper | ¼ to ⅓ cup chicken broth |
| 1 TB. coconut oil | |
| 1 red onion, thinly sliced | |

1. Slice pork loin thinly, and season with caraway seeds, sea salt, and black pepper.

2. Heat a large sauté pan over medium-high heat. Add coconut oil when hot.

3. Add pork loin and brown slightly.

4. Add red onions and porcini mushrooms, and continue to sauté until porcini mushrooms are brown and red onions are slightly translucent.

5. Add red bell peppers, garlic, and chicken broth. Simmer until vegetables are tender and pork is fully cooked (about 20 minutes), and serve hot.

# Beef Pot Roast

Robust and hearty! This meal is easy with a little planning ahead.

| Yield: | Prep time: | Cook time: | Serving size: |
|---|---|---|---|
| 2 lb. roast and 2 cups vegetables | 20 minutes | 3 to 6 hours | 8 oz. roast and ½ cup vegetables |
| **Each serving has:** | | | |
| 509 calories | 14 g carbohydrates | 22 g fat | 64 g protein |

½ tsp. freshly ground black pepper

1 TB. thyme

½ tsp. oregano

1 TB. sea salt (optional)

1 (2- to 3-lb.) lean beef pot roast, rump roast, or chuck shoulder

2 TB. coconut oil

2 yellow onions, sliced

3 carrots, sliced

2 celery stalks, diced

1 bay leaf

3 cups water

1. Mix pepper, thyme, oregano, and sea salt (if using) together in a small bowl.

2. Rub mixture into roast on all sides.

3. Heat a medium skillet (if cooking in a slow cooker) or heavy bottomed oven-proof pan (if cooking in the oven) over high heat. Add coconut oil when hot.

4. Sear all sides of roast.

5. Put roast in a slow cooker, add yellow onions, carrots, celery, bay leaf, and water, and cook until tender, about 4 to 6 hours. Or preheat oven to 325°F, add yellow onions, carrots, celery, bay leaf, and water to the heavy-bottomed, oven-proof pan with meat and roast for 2 to 3 hours until tender.

6. Dish mixture together onto a plate and serve hot.

# Bison Chili

Ground bison is the perfect accompaniment to the spice in this chili.

| Yield: | Prep time: | Cook time: | Serving size: |
|---|---|---|---|
| 6 cups | 10 minutes | 60 to 90 minutes | 1½ cups |
| **Each serving has:** | | | |
| 412 calories | 10 g carbohydrates | 9 g fat | 45 g protein |

1 TB. coconut oil

½ medium yellow onion, diced

3 stalks celery, diced

2 cloves garlic, sliced

1¾ lb. ground bison

2 tsp. ground cumin

2 tsp. thyme

2 tsp. chili powder

1 (12-oz.) jar salsa

1 (8-oz.) can diced tomatoes

1 (7-oz.) can mild green chiles

2 tsp. sea salt

1. Heat a heavy-bottomed soup pot over medium-high heat. When the pan is hot, add coconut oil.

2. Add yellow onion, celery, and garlic and sauté until yellow onions are translucent, about 3 or 4 minutes.

3. Add ground bison, cumin, thyme, and chili powder.

4. Stir while chili cooks, about 5 to 6 minutes.

5. Add salsa, tomatoes, green chiles, and sea salt.

6. Simmer for at least 1 hour. Serve.

**PALEO COMPASS**

Using wild game, such as bison, elk, or venison, is a great way to add a unique flavor to recipes. They are often grass-fed, leaner cuts, and from smaller producers, further increasing their reputation as a healthier option.

# Lamb with Sweet Red Peppers

The warm flavor of cloves with robust lamb is sure to be a favorite on a cold day.

| Yield: | Prep time: | Cook time: | Serving size: |
|---|---|---|---|
| 1 lb. lamb and 4 peppers | 10 minutes | 60 minutes | 4 oz. lamb and 1 pepper |

| Each serving has: | | | |
|---|---|---|---|
| 404 calories | 12 g carbohydrates | 30 g fat | 23 g protein |

1 lb. boneless leg of lamb, cut into 1-in. pieces

½ tsp. sea salt

½ tsp. freshly ground black pepper

3 TB. coconut oil

2 garlic cloves, minced

2 cups hot water

4 large red bell peppers, sliced into rings

3 TB. fresh parsley, chopped

1. Rub lamb pieces with sea salt and black pepper; set aside.

2. Heat a large skillet over high heat and add coconut oil when hot.

3. Brown lamb on all sides, turning frequently, for 3 to 5 minutes.

4. Add garlic and hot water to the pan with lamb, and bring to a boil.

5. Reduce heat to medium, and cook partially covered for 30 minutes.

6. Uncover and cook 10 to 15 minutes longer, or until lamb pieces are tender enough to fall apart with a fork.

7. Add red bell peppers and cook for another 10 minutes, or until peppers are tender.

8. Top with fresh parsley and serve.

# Osso Buco

This recipe boasts concentrated flavors that only develop with its longer cooking time.

| Yield: | Prep time: | Cook time: | Serving size: |
|---|---|---|---|
| 4 veal shanks or 1½ lb. roast | 15 minutes | 2 hours | 6 oz. veal shank or roast |

| Each serving has: | | | |
|---|---|---|---|
| 257 calories | 11 g carbohydrates | 14 g fat | 23 g protein |

4 veal shanks or small veal roast (about 2 lb.)

3 TB. olive oil

Juice of 1 lemon

½ tsp. freshly ground black pepper

1 yellow onion, diced

1 celery stalk, diced

1 medium carrot, diced

1 (14.5-oz.) can diced tomatoes

1 cup water

1. Preheat oven to 350°F.

2. Place veal in single layer in a heavy roasting pan.

3. Sprinkle with olive oil, lemon juice, and pepper. Cover with yellow onion, celery, carrot, and tomatoes.

4. Add water to pan, cover, and roast for 1½ hours or until meat falls off the bone.

5. Uncover and brown for 30 minutes longer, adding hot water if necessary.

6. Transfer to plates and serve hot.

**Variation:** This dish is traditionally topped with Gremolata for extra flavor. You can make your own by mixing minced garlic, fresh parsley, lemon zest, sea salt, and black pepper.

# Slow Cooker Pork Loin

Good things are worth waiting for with this one-pot meal.

| Yield: | Prep time: | Cook time: | Serving size: |
|---|---|---|---|
| 8 cups | 10 minutes | 6 to 7 hours | 2 cups |

| Each serving has: | | | |
|---|---|---|---|
| 331 calories | 19 g carbohydrates | 11 g fat | 41 g protein |

| | |
|---|---|
| 1½ lb. pork loin | 1 head cauliflower, separated into medium-size florets |
| 1 (16-oz.) can tomato sauce | 1 or 2 TB. dried basil |
| 1 medium (6- to 8-in.) zucchini, sliced | Freshly ground black pepper |

1. Place pork, tomato sauce, zucchini, cauliflower, basil, and pepper in a large slow cooker.

2. Cook on low for 6 to 7 hours, or until meat and vegetables are tender. Serve hot.

# Classic Chicken and Turkey

## In This Chapter

- Going tropical with chicken
- Pairing seasonal fruit and turkey
- New burger favorites
- Spicy poultry classics

The labels used to describe the quality of the chicken and turkey you buy can be a little confusing, and sometimes misleading. There's "natural," "organic," "vegetarian diet," and others. What do they mean? The USDA defines "natural" or "all natural" as "a product containing no artificial ingredients or added color and is only minimally processed …." That's it. You have to do your research to find out how the animal lived and what it was eating. "Free range" usually means the animals weren't in cages, but it doesn't guarantee their living conditions were good. Again, you have to do your research. "Organic" means that the birds haven't eaten pesticides or antibiotics, and that their quality of life is monitored by the USDA's limited resources. Organic is usually better than free range or all natural, and "pasture raised from a local farm" is the most Paleo of all.

In this chapter, we explore some recipes that go way beyond a typical roasted chicken breast. We start off with quick recipes, like Cilantro Turkey Burgers and Grilled Chicken with Rosemary and Bacon, and then progress to more time-consuming recipes that are well worth the effort, like Chicken Cacciatore.

# Cilantro Turkey Burgers

Fresh cilantro and crisp red onion make these burgers a real treat any time of the year. This easy alternative to beef burgers may soon become your new favorite—and you won't even miss the bun! Serve with a side dish for a complete meal.

| Yield: | Prep time: | Cook time: | Serving size: |
|---|---|---|---|
| 4 (4-oz.) patties | 10 minutes | 10 minutes | 2 (4-oz.) patties |
| **Each serving has:** | | | |
| 287 calories | 4 g carbohydrates | 5 g fat | 57 g protein |

| | |
|---|---|
| 1 lb. ground turkey | 1 tsp. sea salt |
| 1 cup cilantro, chopped | ¼ tsp. freshly ground black pepper |
| ¼ cup red onion, finely chopped | ½ tsp. coconut oil (only used if broiling) |
| 2 tsp. garlic, minced | |

1. Prepare the grill or turn the broiler on low.

2. Combine turkey, cilantro, red onion, and garlic in a bowl, using a fork to mix well.

3. Shape into 4 patties. Sprinkle with sea salt and pepper.

4. Grill or broil until inner temperature is at least 165°F. Note: if broiling, grease pan lightly with coconut oil to prevent sticking.

5. Serve hot with your choice of condiments.

**Variation:** Use ground dark meat turkey or chicken for a little more flavor.

# Coconut Chicken

This mild recipe is perfect for those who dislike potent flavors.

| Yield: | Prep time: | Cook time: | Serving size: |
|---|---|---|---|
| 4 chicken breasts | 10 minutes | 10 minutes | 1 chicken breast |

| Each serving has: | | | |
|---|---|---|---|
| 347 calories | 7 g carbohydrates | 24 g fat | 31 g protein |

½ cup almond flour

½ cup unsweetened shredded coconut

¼ tsp. sea salt

1 egg

1 lb. boneless, skinless chicken breasts

2 TB. coconut oil

1. Mix almond flour, shredded coconut, and sea salt together in a bowl.

2. Beat egg in a separate bowl.

3. Dip each chicken breast in egg and then coat in dry mixture.

4. Heat a frying pan over medium-high heat and add coconut oil when hot.

5. Pan-fry chicken breasts until fully cooked, or until juices run clear and there is no pink in the middle. Serve.

**DAMAGE CONTROL**

With chicken, it's especially important to make sure you cook the meat thoroughly. The USDA recommends cooking chicken to an internal temperature of 165°F to reduce exposure to food-borne illness. To keep chicken juicy, remove from heat when internal temperature reaches 160°F and let rest until a safe temperature is reached. Also, it is important to not use wooden cutting boards when handling raw chicken since they can retain bacteria, and to be aware of cross-contamination in your kitchen prep area.

# Grilled Chicken with Rosemary and Bacon

Rosemary and bacon add a distinct punch in this meal to dress up otherwise ordinary chicken.

| Yield: | Prep time: | Cook time: | Serving size: |
|---|---|---|---|
| 4 chicken breasts | 10 minutes | 20 minutes | 1 chicken breast |

| Each serving has: | | | |
|---|---|---|---|
| 186 calories | 3 g carbohydrates | 6 g fat | 30 g protein |

4 (4-oz.) boneless, skinless chicken breasts

4 tsp. garlic powder

½ tsp. sea salt

¼ tsp. freshly ground black pepper

4 sprigs fresh rosemary

4 thick slices bacon

4 toothpicks (optional)

1. Season chicken breasts with garlic powder, sea salt, and pepper.

2. Lay 1 rosemary sprig on top of each chicken breast and wrap 1 slice of bacon around to hold rosemary in place. Secure each piece of bacon with a toothpick (if using) or another rosemary sprig.

3. Grill chicken breasts about 8 minutes per side, or until juices run clear and there is no pink in the middle, and bacon is fully cooked. Serve.

**Variation:** For a more exotic dish, replace chicken breasts with split-breast, bone-in Cornish game hens.

# Grilled Chicken Kebabs with Garlic and Cumin

These fragrant kebabs are not shy on garlic!

| Yield: | Prep time: | Cook time: | Serving size: |
|---|---|---|---|
| 16 kebabs | 2¼ hours | 20 minutes | 4 kebabs |

| Each serving has: | | | |
|---|---|---|---|
| 392 calories | 6 g carbohydrates | 17 g fat | 52 g protein |

| | |
|---|---|
| 1 lb. boneless, skinless chicken breasts | 2 TB. sesame oil |
| 2 cloves garlic, crushed | ½ tsp. sea salt |
| 2 TB. ground cumin | Wooden skewers |

1. Slice chicken breasts lengthwise into 3 or 4 strips each.

2. Combine crushed garlic, cumin, sesame oil, and sea salt in a bowl.

3. Place chicken into spice mixture and coat each piece. Cover and refrigerate for 2 hours.

4. Just before dinnertime, prepare the grill at medium-high heat and soak the skewers in water for at least 15 minutes to prevent burning.

5. Pierce each slice of chicken breast with a skewer.

6. Grill chicken until fully cooked, about 6 to 8 minutes per side, or until juices run clear and there is no pink in the middle. Serve hot or eat cold as leftovers.

**PALEO COMPASS**

Try pairing this recipe with Mojo Verde for a spicy kick (recipe in Chapter 12).

# Apple-Glazed Turkey Breasts

The tarragon in this dish is a surprisingly good match with the apple juice and fresh ginger.

| Yield: | Prep time: | Cook time: | Serving size: |
|---|---|---|---|
| 4 turkey cutlets | 10 minutes | 30 minutes | 1 turkey cutlet |

| Each serving has: | | | |
|---|---|---|---|
| 168 calories | 6 g carbohydrates | 4 g fat | 25 g protein |

½ cup apple juice (or the juice of 1 medium/large apple)

½ cup chicken stock

2 cloves garlic, minced

4 TB. fresh tarragon, minced

1 tsp. fresh ginger, grated

4 (4- to 6-oz.) turkey breast cutlets

¼ tsp. sea salt (optional)

¼ tsp. freshly ground black pepper (optional)

1 TB. coconut oil

1. Combine apple juice, chicken stock, garlic, tarragon, and ginger together in a small bowl. Set aside.

2. Season both sides of turkey cutlets with sea salt (if using) and pepper (if using).

3. Heat a large skillet over medium-high heat. When pan is hot, add coconut oil.

4. Sear each cutlet 1 to 2 minutes on each side, until browned. Place on plate and set aside.

5. Reduce heat to medium and add apple juice mixture to pan.

6. As sauce comes to a boil, return turkey cutlets to the pan. Simmer until sauce reduces and turkey is fully cooked (about 20 to 25 minutes). Serve.

# Chicken and Sweet Potatoes with Shallots

Sweet, savory, and all-around delicious!

| Yield: | Prep time: | Cook time: | Serving size: |
|---|---|---|---|
| 4 chicken breasts and 4 cups potatoes | 15 minutes | 45 minutes | 1 chicken breast and 1 cup potatoes |
| **Each serving has:** | | | |
| 295 calories | 13 g carbohydrates | 15 g fat | 27 g protein |

1½ lb. (about 4 medium) sweet potatoes, peeled and cut in 2-in. pieces

1½ tsp. sea salt

4 (4- to 6-oz.) boneless, skinless chicken breasts

¼ tsp. freshly ground black pepper

4 TB. coconut oil

4 shallots, sliced into ¼-in. rings

2 TB. fresh rosemary, chopped

1. Place sweet potatoes in a large pot and cover with cold water.

2. Bring pot to a boil. Once boiling, add 1 teaspoon sea salt and reduce heat to medium-low. Simmer until tender, about 14 to 16 minutes.

3. Reserve ¼ cup of cooking water. Drain remaining liquid and return sweet potatoes to pot. Mash with reserved cooking water and set aside.

4. Season chicken with remaining ½ teaspoon sea salt and pepper.

5. Heat coconut oil in a large skillet over medium-high heat.

6. When pan is hot, add sliced shallots and rosemary and cook for a minute.

7. Add chicken breasts to pan and pan-fry until golden brown and fully cooked, 7 to 8 minutes per side.

8. Serve with mashed sweet potatoes on the side.

# Grilled Chicken Mediterranean

The bold flavors of this dish stand out even when served cold as leftovers.

| Yield: | Prep time: | Cook time: | Serving size: |
|---|---|---|---|
| 4 chicken breasts | 10 minutes | 30 minutes | 1 chicken breast |

| Each serving has: | | | |
|---|---|---|---|
| 219 calories | 5 g carbohydrates | 10 g fat | 27 g protein |

| | |
|---|---|
| 1 cup cherry or grape tomatoes | 4 (4- to 6-oz.) boneless, skinless chicken breasts |
| 16 to 18 large kalamata olives, pitted and halved | ½ tsp. sea salt |
| 3 TB. capers, rinsed | ¼ tsp. freshly ground black pepper |
| 6 tsp. olive oil | |

1. Preheat oven to 475°F.

2. Toss cherry tomatoes, kalamata olives, capers, and 2 teaspoons olive oil in a bowl.

3. Season chicken breasts on both sides with sea salt and pepper.

4. Heat a large, oven-proof skillet over high heat. Once hot, add 2 teaspoons olive oil and sear chicken on both sides.

5. Reduce heat to medium-high and add remaining 2 teaspoons olive oil (should be hot but not smoking) and continue to cook until deep golden brown, about 4 minutes.

6. Use tongs to flip chicken and then add tomato mixture to skillet.

7. Transfer skillet to the oven and roast chicken until cooked through and tomatoes have softened, about 15 to 18 minutes.

8. Transfer to the plates and spoon tomato mixture over top to serve.

**Variation:** Try using skin-on chicken breasts to give the meat a crisp and more savory topping.

# Honey-Walnut Chicken

This dish has sweetness from the honey and nutty flavors from the walnuts, making it a showstopper.

| Yield: | Prep time: | Cook time: | Serving size: |
|---|---|---|---|
| 4 chicken breasts | 10 minutes | 25 minutes | 1 chicken breast |

| Each serving has: | | | |
|---|---|---|---|
| 270 calories | 14 g carbohydrates | 13 g fat | 28 g protein |

| | |
|---|---|
| 1 TB. olive oil | ½ cup walnuts, chopped |
| 1 TB. fresh thyme | ⅓ cup apple cider vinegar |
| 1 tsp. sea salt | 3 TB. raw honey |
| ¼ tsp. freshly ground black pepper | ½ cup water |
| 4 (4- to 6-oz.) boneless, skinless chicken breasts | |

1. Combine olive oil, thyme, sea salt, and pepper.

2. Rub chicken breasts with seasoning and set aside while preparing other ingredients.

3. In a 12-inch nonstick skillet, toast walnuts over medium-low heat for 4 to 6 minutes or until golden and fragrant, stirring constantly. Note: walnuts will burn quickly if left unattended.

4. Transfer walnuts to a dish, and turn heat up to medium under the hot skillet.

5. Add chicken to the same skillet. Cook 12 minutes or until done, turning frequently.

6. Transfer chicken to a clean plate, keeping drippings in the skillet.

7. Add apple cider vinegar to chicken drippings in the hot skillet and cook for 1 minute, stirring constantly.

8. Add raw honey and water, and simmer 6 to 7 minutes until slightly thickened. Stir in walnuts and serve on top of chicken.

**PALEO COMPASS**

Raw honey and coconut sap are the best Paleo sweeteners. They have low glycemic indexes and high nutrient concentrations. However, maple syrup is an acceptable alternative in a pinch. It has a higher glycemic index but offers a wide array of nutrients like magnesium and iron.

# Roast Chicken with Balsamic Bell Peppers

The balsamic vinegar in this dish adds zing!

| Yield: | Prep time: | Cook time: | Serving size: |
|---|---|---|---|
| 4 chicken breasts with peppers | 10 minutes | 35 minutes | 1 chicken breast with peppers |

| Each serving has: | | | |
|---|---|---|---|
| 224 calories | 11 g carbohydrates | 9 g fat | 28 g protein |

1¼ tsp. sea salt (optional)

¾ tsp. freshly ground black pepper

¾ tsp. fennel seeds, crushed

¼ tsp. garlic powder

¼ tsp. dried oregano

4 (4- to 6-oz.) skinless, boneless
    chicken breasts

6 tsp. olive oil

1 large shallot, thinly sliced

2 tsp. fresh rosemary, chopped

2 red bell peppers, thinly sliced

1 yellow bell pepper, thinly sliced

1 cup chicken broth

1 TB. balsamic vinegar

1. Preheat oven to 450°F.

2. Combine 1 teaspoon sea salt (if using), ½ teaspoon black pepper, fennel seeds, garlic powder, and oregano.

3. Brush chicken breasts with 2 teaspoons olive oil and sprinkle spice rub over chicken.

4. Heat a large skillet over medium-high heat and add 2 teaspoons olive oil.

5. Add chicken and cook 3 minutes or until browned. Turn each piece and cook 1 minute more.

6. Remove chicken from pan and arrange in a large baking dish. Bake for 15 to 20 minutes, or until fully cooked.

7. Meanwhile, heat remaining 2 teaspoons oil over medium-high heat in the same large skillet used to brown chicken (do not wash it first).

8. When the pan is hot, add shallots and rosemary, and sauté 3 to 5 minutes, or until shallots are translucent.

9. Add red bell peppers and yellow bell peppers, and stir in chicken broth, scraping the pan to loosen brown bits.

10. Reduce heat and simmer 5 minutes. Add balsamic vinegar and season with remaining ¼ teaspoon sea salt (if using) and remaining ¼ teaspoon black pepper. Cook 3 minutes more, stirring frequently.

11. Serve sauce over chicken.

# Turkey Vegetable Meatballs

These meatballs are so good you may find yourself eating leftovers for breakfast or a snack.

| Yield: | Prep time: | Cook time: | Serving size: |
|---|---|---|---|
| 12 to 20 meatballs | 10 minutes | 30 minutes | 3 to 5 meatballs |
| **Each serving has:** | | | |
| 200 calories | 12 g carbohydrates | 8 g fat | 25 g protein |

| | |
|---|---|
| 2 medium carrots (or handful of baby carrots) | 2 tsp. garlic salt |
| 1 red or green bell pepper, seeded | ½ cup fresh parsley |
| 5 large white button mushrooms | 2 TB. Italian seasoning |
| ½ yellow onion | ½ tsp. freshly ground black pepper |
| 1 clove garlic | 1 lb. ground turkey or chicken |

1. Preheat oven to 350°F.

2. Place carrots, red bell pepper, mushrooms, yellow onion, garlic, garlic salt, parsley, Italian seasoning, and black pepper in a food processor and blend until well chopped.

3. Empty the food processor into a large bowl, add ground turkey, and mix together completely.

4. Form meatballs (about 1½ to 2 inches each) and place on a nongreased baking sheet. Bake for about 25 minutes, or until completely cooked. Serve hot or cold.

# Teriyaki Chicken

With sweet onions, peppers, and pineapple, you'll have plenty of sweetness without the added sugar found in a traditional Western version of this dish.

| Yield: | Prep time: | Cook time: | Serving size: |
|---|---|---|---|
| 4 (4-oz.) chicken breasts | 10 minutes | 25 minutes | 1 chicken breast |
| **Each serving has:** | | | |
| 208 calories | 14 g carbohydrates | 6 g fat | 28 g protein |

1 lb. boneless, skinless chicken
   breasts
¼ tsp. sea salt
¼ tsp. freshly ground black pepper
1 TB. coconut oil
1 medium yellow onion, diced

2 TB. coconut aminos
1 cup pineapple, diced (fresh or
   canned in juice)
1 medium red bell pepper, diced
3 romaine lettuce hearts, chopped

1. Cut chicken breasts into 1-inch pieces and season lightly with sea salt and black pepper.

2. Heat a large skillet over medium-high heat and add coconut oil when hot.

3. Add yellow onions and chicken to the pan and cook about 5 minutes.

4. Add coconut aminos and continue to cook another 5 minutes.

5. Add pineapple and red bell peppers and cook until chicken is cooked and vegetables are tender.

6. Serve over chopped romaine lettuce.

**PALEO COMPASS**

Coconut aminos, made from raw coconut tree sap, are an excellent replacement for tamari or soy sauce. They contain high amounts of amino acids and leave out the wheat and soy found in soy sauce. They can be found online or at most health food markets, such as Whole Foods.

# Thai Chicken Wraps

This recipe is all about the nutty Thai sauce.

| Yield: | Prep time: | Cook time: | Serving size: |
|---|---|---|---|
| 8 lettuce wraps | 20 minutes | 20 minutes | 2 lettuce wraps |
| **Each serving has:** | | | |
| 259 calories | 14 g carbohydrates | 10 g fat | 32 g protein |

¼ cup almond butter

¼ cup water

2 TB. coconut aminos

2 TB. lime juice (or the juice of 1 lime)

2 cloves garlic, minced

1 lb. boneless, skinless chicken breasts

1 cup raw broccoli, finely chopped

4 Napa cabbage leaves, thinly chopped

1 large carrot, shredded

3 green onions, thinly sliced

¼ cup fresh cilantro

8 Bibb or romaine lettuce leaves

1. For Thai sauce, whisk together almond butter, water, coconut aminos, lime juice, and garlic. Set aside.

2. Grill chicken breasts and dice into ½-inch cubes.

3. Combine chicken, broccoli, Napa cabbage, carrots, green onions, and cilantro.

4. Wash lettuce leaves and spread out on a plate. (Reserve half the leaves for leftovers.)

5. Fill plated lettuce leaves with chicken mixture. Drizzle with Thai sauce and serve.

6. Reserve leftover filling mixture for lunch the next day, but wait to fill lettuce leaves until serving so lettuce stays crisp.

# Chicken Cacciatore

Just like your grandmother used to make … except better for you!

| Yield: | Prep time: | Cook time: | Serving size: |
|---|---|---|---|
| 32 oz. chicken and 3 cups vegetables | 15 minutes | 55 minutes | 6 oz. chicken and ½ cup vegetables |

| Each serving has: | | | |
|---|---|---|---|
| 336 calories | 17 g carbohydrates | 19 g fat | 26 g protein |

3 TB. olive or coconut oil

1 (3-lb.) bone-in chicken, cut up

½ tsp. sea salt

½ tsp. freshly ground black pepper

1 medium yellow onion, sliced

½ lb. white button mushrooms, sliced

3 cloves garlic, minced

1 (16-oz.) can diced tomatoes

1 (8-oz.) can tomato sauce

1 tsp. dried oregano

1 large green bell pepper, cut into 1-in. pieces

1. In a large skillet, heat olive oil over medium-high heat.

2. Season chicken with sea salt and black pepper.

3. When pan is hot, add chicken and brown on all sides, about 10 minutes.

4. Remove chicken pieces and let drain on paper towels.

5. Add yellow onions and mushrooms to the hot pan and sauté until onions are slightly translucent, about 5 minutes.

6. Add garlic, tomatoes, tomato sauce, oregano, and green bell pepper. Stir well.

7. Return chicken to the pan and bring to a boil.

8. Once boiling, reduce heat, cover, and simmer 30 minutes, until chicken is tender. Serve hot.

# Curry Chicken and Cauliflower Rice

Exploding with flavor, this meal is another favorite to share with your non-Paleo friends.

| Yield: | Prep time: | Cook time: | Serving size: |
|---|---|---|---|
| 1 lb. chicken breasts and 6 cups vegetables | 35 minutes | 45 minutes | 4 oz. chicken breast and 1½ cups vegetables |
| **Each serving has:** | | | |
| 368 calories | 23 g carbohydrates | 19 g fat | 31 g protein |

1 TB. ginger root, finely minced or grated

1 clove garlic, minced

1 TB. ground cumin

1 tsp. ground coriander

½ tsp. plus dash cayenne pepper

¼ tsp. ground cardamom

½ tsp. ground cloves

1½ tsp. sea salt

¾ tsp. freshly ground black pepper

3 TB. coconut oil

1 lb. boneless, skinless chicken breasts

6 white button mushrooms, sliced

1 (13.6-oz.) can unsweetened coconut milk

2 TB. lemon juice

1 large (10- to 12-in.) zucchini, diced

1 red bell pepper, diced

1 medium-size head of cauliflower

½ tsp. ground curry powder

1 green onion, finely chopped

4 TB. fresh cilantro, chopped

1 small cucumber, diced

¼ red onion, diced

1. Mix ginger root, garlic, cumin, coriander, ¼ teaspoon cayenne, cardamom, cloves, 1 teaspoon sea salt, and ½ teaspoon black pepper in a large bowl.

2. Cut chicken breasts into 1-inch pieces and put in the bowl with spices. Coat chicken with spice mixture and set aside.

3. Over medium heat, add 2 tablespoons coconut oil to a large skillet.

4. When hot, add chicken, mushrooms, coconut milk, and lemon juice to the pan. Simmer over medium heat for 15 minutes.

5. Add zucchini and red bell pepper, and continue to cook until chicken is done, about 5 to 10 minutes.

6. While chicken is cooking, prepare cauliflower rice. Wash and rough-chop cauliflower and place in a large skillet with remaining 1 tablespoon coconut oil and cook over medium-high heat until slightly softened and tender.

7. Place softened cauliflower, curry powder, green onion, and remaining dash of cayenne pepper into a food processor and pulse until it has a grainy ricelike consistency. Season with remaining ½ teaspoon sea salt and remaining ¼ teaspoon black pepper.

8. Serve chicken curry over cauliflower rice and garnish with chopped cilantro, cucumber, and red onion.

# Fruited Chicken Thighs

The fruit stuffing adds savory sweetness to this skin-on chicken meal.

| Yield: | Prep time: | Cook time: | Serving size: |
|---|---|---|---|
| 4 chicken thighs | 30 minutes | 60 minutes | 1 chicken thigh |
| **Each serving has:** | | | |
| 559 calories | 24 g carbohydrates | 41 g fat | 27 g protein |

| | |
|---|---|
| 6 TB. olive oil | ¼ cup golden raisins |
| 1 medium yellow onion, diced | ¼ cup walnuts, chopped |
| 1 celery stalk, diced | 1 egg, beaten |
| 1 garlic clove, minced | 4 (6-oz.) chicken thighs, skin on |
| 2 medium apples, cored and diced | 1 tsp. dried tarragon |

1. Preheat oven to 350°F.

2. Heat 2 tablespoons olive oil in a skillet over medium-high heat.

3. When the pan is hot, add yellow onion, celery, and garlic. Sauté about 3 minutes, until onion and celery are tender. Remove from heat.

4. Add apples, golden raisins, walnuts, and egg to onion mixture. Mix well.

5. Prepare chicken thighs by gently pulling the skin away from the meat without removing it.

6. Stuff apple mixture between skin and meat.

7. Arrange chicken pieces in a foil-lined baking dish with skin facing up.

8. In a small bowl, combine remaining 4 tablespoons olive oil with tarragon. Brush over chicken thighs.

9. Bake, uncovered, basting every 15 minutes, for 1 hour or until chicken is fully cooked.

**Variation:** Use duck breast instead of chicken thighs for a special occasion dish.

# Spiced Chicken with Peaches and Pineapple Sauce

Nutty, sweet, and spicy, this recipe has a flavor that appeals to everyone.

| Yield: | Prep time: | Cook time: | Serving size: |
|---|---|---|---|
| 32 oz. chicken and 3 cups fruit | 15 minutes | 65 minutes | 6 oz. chicken and ½ cup fruit |

| Each serving has: | | | |
|---|---|---|---|
| 391 calories | 42 g carbohydrates | 13 g fat | 27 g protein |

1 (3-lb.) bone-in chicken, cut up

1 (8-oz.) can crushed pineapple in juice

1 cup orange juice with no added sweetener

½ cup raisins

½ cup sliced almonds

¼ tsp. cinnamon

¼ tsp. ground cloves

1 lb. (3 to 4 medium peaches), sliced and puréed; frozen or canned may be used (if using canned, rinse and drain well)

Freshly ground black pepper

Sea salt

1. In a large skillet, combine chicken, pineapple, orange juice, raisins, almonds, cinnamon, and cloves.

2. Simmer partly covered for 45 minutes, turning chicken occasionally.

3. Add peach purée to pan and stir.

4. Simmer uncovered 15 minutes longer, until chicken is tender and sauce is slightly thickened.

5. Season to taste with pepper and sea salt and serve.

# Delectable Desserts

## In This Chapter

- Good-for-you cookies
- Muffins, cakes, and tarts, Paleo style
- No-bake apple pie
- A double helping of ice cream

A new diet wouldn't be complete without desserts! The occasional dessert helps keep you compliant by assuaging your sweet tooth. While the cookies, cakes, tarts, and ice cream in this chapter are much better for you than the white flour, refined sugar, and pasteurized dairy used in conventional desserts, they're still higher in sugar than the typical Paleo meal. So if you're trying to lose weight, keep them to a minimum—say, once a week or so.

The source of sweetness in Paleo desserts is usually raw honey, but sometimes maple syrup, fruit juice, dates, or other dried fruit is used. The flours most often used are coconut flour, almond flour, and occasionally tapioca flour. And the usual butter and milk are replaced by coconut oil, coconut milk, and nut butters. Recipes occasionally call for chocolate and often take advantage of fruit's natural sweetness.

With these simple ingredients, you can make treats that even your non-Paleo friends will love. They won't even have to know you've done them a favor by sparing them the grains and refined sugars. We hope you enjoy your new Almond Macaroons, Grain-Free Chocolate Chip Cookies, Carrot Cake, and many others!

# Almond Macaroons

These delectable treats are light and tasty.

| Yield: | Prep time: | Cook time: | Serving size: |
|---|---|---|---|
| 20 macaroons | 10 minutes | 30 minutes | 3 macaroons |
| **Each serving has:** | | | |
| 320 calories | 21 g carbohydrates | 24 g fat | 12 g protein |

1¼ cups almonds

⅛ tsp. ground cinnamon

2 TB. lemon zest

2 egg whites

¼ cup raw honey

2 TB. lemon juice

1. Preheat oven to 250°F.

2. Line a baking sheet with parchment paper.

3. Grind or chop almonds coarsely. (This could also be done in a food processor, but be sure not to grind into a paste.) Set aside.

4. Mix cinnamon and lemon zest in a medium bowl.

5. Beat egg whites and add to mixture.

6. Add honey and lemon juice and stir vigorously to blend thoroughly.

7. Add almond mixture and blend thoroughly.

8. Use a teaspoon to scoop small portions of batter onto parchment paper.

9. Bake 30 minutes.

10. Remove from the paper with a spatula while still slightly warm and serve.

# Grain-Free Chocolate Chip Cookies

So good, even your kids will love them!

| Yield: | Prep time: | Cook time: | Serving size: |
|---|---|---|---|
| 24 cookies | 25 minutes | 20 minutes | 1 cookie |

| **Each serving has:** | | | |
|---|---|---|---|
| 212 calories | 16 g carbohydrates | 17 g fat | 5 g protein |

3 cups almond flour

1 tsp. baking soda

1 tsp. sea salt

2 large eggs

½ cup raw honey

1 tsp. vanilla extract

½ cup coconut oil, melted (see following sidebar)

1½ cups semi-sweet chocolate chips (no sugar added)

1. Preheat oven to 375°F.

2. Line a baking sheet with parchment paper.

3. In a small bowl, mix almond flour, baking soda, and sea salt. Set aside.

4. In a medium mixing bowl, beat eggs, honey, and vanilla extract with a hand mixer or wire whisk.

5. Pour dry ingredients slowly into wet ingredients as you beat with mixer or mix with a fork until combined.

6. Add melted coconut oil and continue to blend until combined. Stir in chocolate chips.

7. Drop tablespoon-size balls of cookie dough onto prepared baking sheet.

8. Bake for approximately 8 to 10 minutes.

9. Remove from paper with a spatula and let cool. Serve.

**PALEO COMPASS**

If coconut oil gets too cool, it solidifies. You can melt the oil by placing it in a saucepan over low heat.

# Paleo Cookies

These delicious cookies are easy to make!

| Yield: | Prep time: | Cook time: | Serving size: |
| --- | --- | --- | --- |
| 36 cookies | 10 minutes | 35 minutes | 2 cookies |

| Each serving has: | | | |
| --- | --- | --- | --- |
| 351 calories | 39 g carbohydrates | 22 g fat | 5 g protein |

| | |
| --- | --- |
| 2 cups raw honey | ½ tsp. ground ginger |
| 4 cups almond flour | 2 cups walnuts, ground |
| ½ tsp. freshly grated nutmeg | ½ cup dried fruit, chopped |

1. Preheat oven to 350°F.

2. Line a baking sheet with parchment paper.

3. In a small saucepan, warm honey over medium heat. Set aside.

4. Sift together almond flour, nutmeg, and ginger.

5. Pour warm honey into a large mixing bowl and gradually add flour mixture, stirring until well blended.

6. Add walnuts and dried fruit and stir until just combined.

7. Roll dough about ¼ inch thick on a floured board and cut into small squares.

8. Transfer squares to a baking sheet and bake 10 minutes.

9. Remove from paper with a spatula and let cool. Serve.

# Almond Muffins

Follow this recipe exactly for strict Paleo-friendly muffins. If you would like a sweeter taste, add the optional vanilla and coconut sap or raw honey.

| Yield: | Prep time: | Cook time: | Serving size: |
|---|---|---|---|
| 12 muffins | 10 minutes | 15 minutes | 1 muffin |
| **Each serving has:** | | | |
| 314 calories | 13 g carbohydrates | 27 g fat | 9 g protein |

1 cup almond butter

1 cup sliced almonds

1 cup coconut milk

2 cups unsweetened shredded coconut

3 eggs

¼ tsp. vanilla extract (optional)

2 TB. coconut sap or raw honey (optional)

1. Preheat oven to 400°F.

2. Line a muffin tin with paper liners or lightly grease cups with coconut oil.

3. Combine almond butter, sliced almonds, coconut milk, shredded coconut, eggs, vanilla extract (if using), and coconut sap or raw honey (if using) and pour into lined muffin cups.

4. Bake for 15 minutes.

5. Cool muffins before removing from tin and serving.

# Carrot Cake

This dense cake is plenty satisfying even without the traditional frosting.

| Yield: | Prep time: | Cook time: | Serving size: |
| --- | --- | --- | --- |
| 1 (9-in.) cake | 25 minutes | 75 minutes | ⅛ cake |

| Each serving has: | | | |
| --- | --- | --- | --- |
| 398 calories | 30 g carbohydrates | 27 g fat | 14 g protein |

6 eggs, yolks and whites separated

½ cup raw honey (or less if desired)

1½ cups cooked and puréed carrots

1 TB. orange zest

2 TB. unsweetened applesauce

3 cups almond flour

Coconut oil

1. Preheat oven to 325°F.

2. Beat egg yolks and honey together in a medium mixing bowl.

3. Mix in carrot purée, orange zest, applesauce, and almond flour.

4. Using a hand mixer, beat the egg whites in a separate bowl until stiff. Carefully fold into batter.

5. Pour batter into a 9-inch springform pan lightly greased with coconut oil.

6. Bake for about 50 minutes or until a skewer inserted into the cake center comes out clean.

7. Remove from oven and let stand in the pan for 15 minutes, then turn cake out onto a wire rack to cool completely. Serve.

# Paleo Apple Cinnamon Cake

This sweet and spicy cake is an excellent holiday dessert.

| Yield: | Prep time: | Cook time: | Serving size: |
| --- | --- | --- | --- |
| 1 (8-in.) cake | 15 minutes | 30 minutes | ⅛ cake |

| Each serving has: | | | |
| --- | --- | --- | --- |
| 322 calories | 29 g carbohydrates | 22 g fat | 7 g protein |

2 cups almond flour

½ tsp. sea salt

½ tsp. baking soda

¼ cup arrowroot powder (available online, at some farmers' markets, and health food stores)

1 tsp. cinnamon

¼ cup coconut oil, melted

½ cup raw honey

1 egg, beaten

1 TB. vanilla extract (optional)

1 medium apple, peeled, cored, and diced

Coconut oil

Dash freshly grated nutmeg

1. Preheat oven to 350°F.

2. Mix almond flour, sea salt, baking soda, arrowroot powder, and cinnamon in a bowl and stir well to combine.

3. In a separate bowl, stir together coconut oil, honey, egg, and vanilla extract (if using).

4. Stir wet mixture into dry ingredients until just combined. Add apple pieces and stir one more time.

5. Pour batter into a pan greased with coconut oil. Sprinkle with freshly grated nutmeg.

6. For a cake or loaf pan, bake approximately 30 minutes. Let cool and serve.

**PALEO COMPASS**

For an even tastier treat, drizzle raw honey over the cake and serve with Paleo Ice Cream (see recipe later in this chapter). This recipe can also be used to make muffins. For muffins, reduce baking time to 14 minutes.

# Quick and Simple Apple Pie

This no-bake pie is a great version of a fall favorite.

| Yield: | Prep time: | Cook time: | Serving size: |
|---|---|---|---|
| 1 (9-in.) pie | 30 minutes | 60 minutes | ⅛ pie |

| Each serving has: | | | |
|---|---|---|---|
| 230 calories | 48 g carbohydrates | 6 g fat | 3 g protein |

1½ cups sunflower seeds, shelled

¾ cup raisins

1 TB. carob powder

5 to 6 medium-size apples, peeled and cored

1 TB. cinnamon

Juice of ½ lemon

¾ cup raw honey

Dash ground cloves (optional)

¼ cup unsweetened shredded coconut

1. Make pie crust by placing sunflower seeds, raisins, and carob powder in a food processor and process with the *S* blade until finely ground (mixture will stick together).

2. Line a 9-inch pie pan with mixture and form crust.

3. Place apples in food processor and pulse-chop until cut into small pieces. (Be careful not to chop apples too finely and make applesauce.)

4. In a large bowl, combine chopped apples, cinnamon, lemon juice, honey, and cloves (if using).

5. Scoop apple mixture into pie crust. Save the "juice" that remains in the bowl and drizzle over pie when served. Level out with a spatula.

6. Sprinkle shredded coconut on top of pie.

7. Place pie in refrigerator for 1 hour to allow it to set before serving.

**Variation:** Use six ripe peaches instead of apples.

# Baked Banana and Coconut Ice Cream

This puddinglike treat has just the right amount of sweetness.

| Yield: | Prep time: | Cook time: | Serving size: |
|---|---|---|---|
| 2 bananas and 2 scoops ice cream | 5 minutes | 30 minutes | 1 banana and 1 scoop ice cream |

| Each serving has: | | | |
|---|---|---|---|
| 398 calories | 59 g carbohydrates | 21 g fat | 3 g protein |

| | |
|---|---|
| 2 ripe bananas | ½ tsp. ground cinnamon |
| 2 scoops coconut ice cream (store-bought, or see recipe for Paleo Ice Cream later in this chapter) | |

1. Preheat oven to 350°F.

2. Place whole bananas, still in their peel, in an uncovered dish and bake for 20 to 30 minutes until soft.

3. Squeeze out contents of each banana onto two serving plates, and top each banana with scoop of coconut ice cream.

4. Top each with sprinkling of cinnamon and serve.

# Banana, Coconut, and Cashew Cream Tart

This tart looks difficult to make, but it's actually quite easy.

| Yield: | Prep time: | Serving size: | |
|---|---|---|---|
| 1 (9-in.) tart | 30 minutes | ⅛ tart | |
| **Each serving has:** | | | |
| 380 calories | 53 g carbohydrates | 20 g fat | 4 g protein |

1½ cups whole pecans

¼ tsp. sea salt

1½ cups pitted dates

2 TB. raw honey plus 1 TB. (optional)

1 cup raw cashews, soaked overnight and thoroughly drained

½ cup water

1 vanilla bean, split and scraped

¾ cup unsweetened shredded coconut

3 to 4 ripe but firm bananas

1. Coarsely chop pecans in a food processor.

2. Add sea salt and dates, and pulse until thoroughly combined, about 15 to 20 seconds.

3. Add 2 tablespoons raw honey and pulse just until combined. (Mixture should just barely stick together.)

4. Press nut mixture firmly and evenly into a 9-inch pie plate. Set aside.

5. Grind cashews to a coarse paste in a blender.

6. Add water, remaining 1 tablespoon raw honey (if using), and vanilla scrapings, and blend until smooth, about 5 minutes, scraping sides as needed. Mixture should be the consistency of thick pancake batter.

7. Set aside 2 tablespoons shredded coconut; add remainder to blender mixture and process to combine. Pour mixture into prepared pie shell, spreading evenly.

8. Thinly slice bananas and arrange in slightly overlapping rows, beginning at edge of tart.

9. Sprinkle with reserved coconut and serve immediately.

**Variation:** When in season, this tart is excellent with sliced peaches or cut fresh figs instead of bananas.

# Grilled (Pine) Apple and Red Pepper Chutney

This delightful chutney is excellent over ice cream, a small bowl of nuts, or even as a topping for grilled chicken or pork.

| Yield: | Prep time: | Cook time: | Serving size: |
|---|---|---|---|
| 6 cups | 10 minutes | 20 minutes | ½ cup |

| Each serving has: | | | |
|---|---|---|---|
| 229 calories | 60 g carbohydrates | 1 g fat | 2 g protein |

½ tsp. coconut oil

1 (20-oz.) can pineapple rings in juice, drained (or 1 small pineapple, peeled, cored, and cut into rings)

3 Granny Smith apples, cut into rings

1 red bell pepper, diced

1 tsp. cinnamon

½ tsp. sea salt

1. Preheat a griddle over high heat. Add coconut oil.

2. When hot, place pineapple, apples, and red bell pepper onto the griddle.

3. Cook on both sides until fruit gets tender, about 10 to 15 minutes.

4. Remove from heat and chop.

5. Put chopped mixture into a medium skillet and add cinnamon and sea salt.

6. Cook over medium heat for 10 minutes. Serve warm or chilled.

# Paleo Ice Cream

If you have an ice-cream maker, try whipping up a batch of this sweet treat—it makes the perfect summertime dessert.

| Yield: | Prep time: | Cook time: | Serving size: |
|---|---|---|---|
| 4 cups | 5 minutes | 25 minutes | ½ cup |

| Each serving has: | | | |
|---|---|---|---|
| 131 calories | 21 g carbohydrates | 7 g fat | 0 g protein |

| | |
|---|---|
| 2 (13.6-oz.) can coconut milk | Cocoa powder, spices, frozen fruit, nuts, vanilla extract, or other ice-cream flavorings (optional) |
| ½ cup coconut sap (or raw honey) | |

1. Blend coconut milk and coconut sap, along with any additional desired ingredients.

2. Place mixture in an ice-cream maker and wait about 25 minutes. Serve.

**PALEO COMPASS**

The nutritional information provided is for plain ice cream, without additional spices, fruits, or other ingredients.

# Meal Planning

Change can be hard, especially when it involves what you eat. We get stuck in ruts with food because we don't have the time or creativity to make new things. We know that starting a new diet and getting out of those ruts takes a lot of energy, so we want to make it as easy as possible for you.

In this part of the book, you find a four-week meal plan that includes grocery shopping lists. Just take the list to the store every week, buy what's on it, go home and look at the meal plan, and then use the recipes in this book to make your food. If you don't want to follow a meal plan, we describe what your plate should look like to make it Paleo. We also talk about avoiding some common beginner mistakes, calorie counting, and how you might feel in the first couple weeks of the diet.

# Some Practical Advice

## In This Chapter

- What your plate should look like
- Should you count calories?
- Avoiding some common beginner pitfalls
- How you might feel in the beginning

You now understand and appreciate the concept of the diet, and you've even checked out some of the delicious Paleo recipes you might make. But you might still have questions about what your plate should look like if you're not following a recipe to a tee. At some point you're going to improvise, and you'll need to know not only what to cook but how much food to put on your plate.

Portion sizes everywhere have gotten out of hand, making it difficult to know how much is *really* enough. Serving sizes at restaurants and in packaged foods have grown, along with people's weight over the last 20 years. According to the Department of Health and Human Services, a cheeseburger 20 years ago was about 333 calories. Today, a normal cheeseburger is almost twice the size, weighing in at 590 calories! Likewise, typical bagels were 3 inches in diameter 20 years ago, and today they're 6 inches and 350 calories. That's 210 more calories than the bagels of old!

The plates themselves are even bigger nowadays than they used to be, and it's tempting to always fill your plate. Commonly recommended serving sizes can be confusing, and they're often incongruent with the Paleolithic diet, anyway. This chapter should clarify some questions so you can fill your plate properly and avoid making some common newbie mistakes.

# The Paleo Plate

The USDA's "My Plate" guidelines have people believing their plate should be divided into four parts: two big portions for grains and vegetables and two smaller portions for protein and fruits. There's also a bowl on the side (as if a plate weren't big enough for a meal) for low-fat, pasteurized dairy. There's not any mention of fats on the plate, as if to send a subliminal message that they shouldn't be a part of your diet at all. In the fine print, they assure you that vegetable oils should be consumed in modest amounts, but not saturated fats. God forbid.

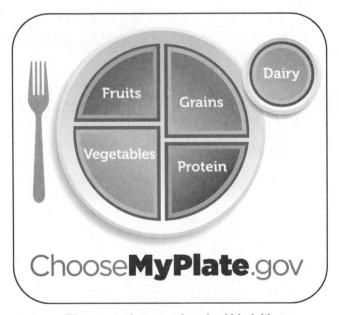

*This is not what your plate should look like.*
(Courtesy of the U.S. Department of Agriculture)

Those guidelines are not what we follow in the Paleo world, as you know by now. Most of what you were likely taught in health class or nutrition class should somehow be extracted from your memory and replaced with more sensible and historically relevant information.

Where the USDA has it wrong is the large portion for grains, the small portion for protein, and omitting fats from the picture.

*Your* plate, which should be considerably smaller than the giant plates you get at big chain restaurants, should be filled with about half plant foods and half animal foods.

Healthy fats should be smattered throughout, either in the form of fat on your meat or added oils and fats. Remember you're aiming for 10 to 40 percent carbs, 20 to 35 percent protein, and 30 to 70 percent fat.

> **PALEO COMPASS**
>
> The percentage ranges of carbohydrates, protein, and fat can be better understood in terms of grams because that's what you normally see on packages and in food charts. For optimal weight loss, you should stay under 100 grams of carbs a day and under 150 grams for weight maintenance, unless you're an endurance athlete. The protein range for normal adults is around 75 to 200 grams per day, and the fat range is 50 to 194 grams per day. The ranges are pretty wide because people's sizes and activity levels vary so much.

Here are a few examples of what your Paleo plate might look like:

- Spinach, onions, and carrots sautéed in coconut oil and a slab of juicy buffalo sirloin

- A big leafy salad topped with almonds, chicken breast, olive oil, lemon juice, and apples

- Roasted pork loin and baked sweet potato with coconut milk drizzled on top

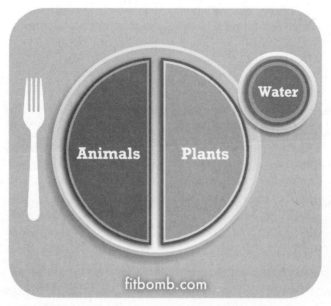

*The picture of your plate would look more like this.*
(Courtesy of Henry Fong of fitbomb.com)

## Portion Sizes

How much of each of the food groups to put on your plate depends on your size and activity level. If you're a 5-foot, 3-inch-tall sedentary woman trying to lose weight, you'd want to eat significantly less than your active, 5-foot, 10-inch husband. However, if you're a fit 5-foot, 3-inch woman working out six times a week on top of being a busy mom, you may need to eat as much as him if he's not that active.

There are, of course, some parameters for serving sizes per meal to help you navigate your plate:

- **Meat, chicken, and fish:** 4 to 8 ounces before cooking
- **Nonstarchy veggies:** 1 to 4 cups raw or ½ to 2 cups cooked
- **Starchy veggies (sweet potatoes, squash, etc.):** ½ to 1½ cups cooked
- **Fruits:** ½ to 2 medium pieces raw; 1 to 2 ounces dried
- **Oils and fats:** 1 teaspoon to 1½ tablespoons
- **Nuts and seeds (includes their respective butters):** 1 to 2 ounces nuts or seeds; 1 to 2 tablespoons nut or seed butter

**PALEO COMPASS**

You can usually buy almond butter or cashew butter in health food stores. Tahini is sesame seed butter, and it can be a fantastic addition to salad dressings or dips.

## Portion Size Translation

But what do all those ounces, teaspoons, and cups look like on your plate? Should you go out and buy a food scale and start measuring everything? No. You're told by the government and conventional medical establishments how much to eat in totally incomprehensible measurements all the time: we don't want you to be confused by this book, too. The truth is that not many people besides professional chefs can precisely portion out a 6-ounce steak or 1 single ounce of almonds. Let's break the confusion down.

### Meat, Chicken, and Seafood

Remember that 16 ounces is 1 pound, so if you go to the store and buy a pound of ground beef and split it up into 4 burgers, you have 4-ounce burgers. Split that raw meat up into 3 equal parts and you have a little more than a 5-ounce burger on your hands (literally).

- 1 ounce is about 3 tablespoons of meat or poultry.

- 2 ounces of meat is a small chicken drumstick or thigh.

- 3 ounces of meat is the size of a deck of cards, a bar of soap, or an average adult's palm.

- 3 ounces of fish is the size of a checkbook.

## Nonstarchy Veggies

This includes leafy vegetables like kale, lettuce, and spinach. Also in this category are peppers, carrots, onions, tomatoes, and even beets and jicama.

- 1 cup of chopped, raw vegetables is the size of a baseball or an average adult's fist.

- ½ cup of cooked vegetables is the size of a billiard ball.

**NUTRITION FACT**

People who switch over to eating Paleo are often concerned they won't get their fiber requirements met without whole grains. Never fear! Calorie for calorie, nonstarchy vegetables are a whopping eight times higher than whole grains in soluble fiber, according to a study done by Dr. Loren Cordain. In his research, he analyzed a sample Paleolithic diet menu (much like the meal plan found in Chapter 18) and found it provided 42.5 grams of fiber, which is higher than the 21 to 38 grams recommended by the USDA. We found very similar results in our comparison of the Paleolithic diet and the Western diet in Appendix E.

## Starchy Veggies

Sweet potatoes, squash, and potatoes are all in the starchy veggie category, among other less well-known foods like taro and plantain.

- 1 medium sweet potato or potato is the size of a computer mouse.

- ½ of a cooked sweet potato is the size of ½ a baseball.

## Fruits

Don't forget that avocados are fruits!

- ½ cup of raw, canned, or frozen fruit is the size of a billiard ball.

- 1 "piece" is the size of a tennis ball.

- ¼ cup or 1 ounce of dried fruit (raisins, prunes, mangoes, etc.) is the size of an egg.

### Oils and Fats

This gets a little tricky when you're pouring oil onto a pan to sauté some veggies. It's hard to tell exactly how much you're serving up. Just once or twice, fill a teaspoon or tablespoon with oil or fat and put it in your pan. Take note of how far out the oil spreads and how it looks in the pan and remember it for the next time you're eyeballing it.

- 1 teaspoon of fat is the size of one die or the tip of a woman's thumb.
- 1 tablespoon is 3 teaspoons.

### Nuts and Seeds

Keep in mind that a little goes a long way with nuts. Even a handful will tide you over for a while because they're so calorie dense.

- 1 ounce of nuts is about a large handful, and that's usually what the serving size is on packaged nuts. 1 ounce is about 23 almonds or 18 cashews.
- 2 tablespoons of nut butter is the size of a ping-pong ball.
- ⅓ cup of nuts is a level handful.

# To Count or Not to Count Calories

If you're trying to lose weight, one of the first things you're normally told to do is count your calories. The only problem is that counting calories can be a real pain in the butt. Not to mention unsustainable. It's time-consuming, tedious, and can be a source of self-judgment. If it goes too far, you might find yourself no longer eating and enjoying food, but instead consuming calories and accordingly labeling yourself good or bad.

That's not to say that it doesn't work. Calorie counting can be very useful if you're trying to lose weight, but so can the Paleolithic diet. People are often overweight because they eat too many refined carbohydrates, which leads to sugar "buzzes" and blood sugar crashes, throughout every day. The crashes create cravings and the cravings lead to overconsuming high glycemic foods like grains, legumes, and refined sugars: it's a vicious cycle.

The Paleolithic diet, and in particular, the meal plan we provide in Chapter 18, help solve those issues. You're eating breakfast, lunch, a snack, and dinner every day and each is complete with high-quality protein, fat, and carbohydrates, so your blood sugar doesn't have a chance to spike or plummet. That means fewer sugar cravings and less overconsumption. Problem solved.

Usually when people eat Paleo, they lose weight without counting calories. The diet is a relief for your body, and it curbs hunger. Body weight normalizes to its natural state, whether that means gaining weight in the form of muscle or losing body fat or both.

If you're trying to lose weight, start off by following the plan and not counting calories. If you don't lose any weight after about a month, have an honest chat with yourself about whether or not you *actually* followed the plan. It's easy to sneak in some bread here, some cookies or cake there, and a beer every night.

If you decide that you've been incredibly dedicated to the diet and you're still not losing weight, investigate the amount of food you're eating (without counting calories just yet). For instance, if you're feeling weak throughout the day, like you don't have enough fuel in your system, then you're not getting enough food. Sometimes not eating enough can put your body into "starvation mode": your body perceives the lack of food as a threat and it holds onto fat just in case you don't eat for a while. It's an evolutionary thing. On the other hand, if you're feeling stuffed and bloated every time you eat, then you're obviously eating too much. Adjust your portions as necessary.

If all that doesn't work, and you still aren't losing weight, consider counting calories. But how do you do it? There are free online tools like fitday.com and myfitnesspal.com that help you figure out, according to your size and activity level, how much you should be eating and how much you *are* eating. You can input your statistics and the program will provide a target calorie goal. Then you enter all the foods you eat every day, as well as your exercise, to find out whether you're high or low in calories. The program usually puts you on target to lose 1 or 2 pounds per week, which is a healthy goal.

One thing to be aware of is that those programs' suggestions for carbohydrate, protein, and fat intake are usually discordant with the Paleolithic diet because they're based on the USDA's dietary recommendations. Go with your new knowledge about the detriments of high carbohydrate intake and the benefits of higher fat and protein intake, and disregard their recommendations.

**PALEO COMPASS**

People are very different in their ability to burn the calories they've eaten in exercise and everyday activities, so using online tools to calculate your caloric needs is not an exact science. Two people of the same age, gender, height, weight, and even the same level of fitness can burn a different number of calories doing the exact same exercise. For instance, if the average number of calories burned by walking briskly for 15 minutes is 100, people will burn anywhere from 70 to 130 calories.

If you end up counting calories, we suggest you do it for long enough to get to know how much food keeps you losing or maintaining your weight. Then stop counting and see if you can let your body be your guide. Trust that you'll know when to eat and when you've had enough. Your body is wiser than you might think!

Also keep in mind that body weight can fluctuate quite a bit day to day, depending on hydration, menstrual cycles, and other factors, so try not to weigh yourself every day. You may gain a pound one day and lose several pounds the next. In order to avoid unnecessary disappointment, get on the scale not more than once a week to see what your cumulative loss is.

# Avoiding Common Mistakes

Rookies don't always get it right, and that's okay. But you can learn from other Paleo newbies' mistakes to get the most out of the diet quickly. The following are some common blunders people make that challenge their commitment to the diet in the beginning. Don't let them happen to you.

## Skimping on Carbohydrates

Yes, Paleo can be a low-carbohydrate diet, and low-carb diets are good for losing weight, but there's no need to forgo all carbs at any point in the diet to hastily increase weight loss. This isn't Atkins. A lot of people aren't used to eating as many vegetables as it takes to get those 100ish grams of carbs a day. If you start to go below 50 grams of carbs every day (for reference, a medium apple contains about 21 grams and one bunch of spinach has 12), you can go into ketosis. Ketosis isn't necessarily a bad thing—it just means you use fat as your primary fuel instead of carbohydrates. The problem is that ketosis can feel pretty bad, especially in the beginning when your body is adapting to the change.

If you feel like you're walking through oatmeal throughout the day—slow, tired, sluggish—you may not be getting enough carbohydrates. Eat more fruits and vegetables, and if you're active, eat more starchy carbs.

## Fearing the Fat

Alternatively, you can increase the fat in your diet if you're having those lethargic symptoms. Your body is very good at turning fat into energy and will not necessarily make you fat, despite the "eating fat makes you fat" myth. Yes, if you eat a lot of fat *and* a lot of carbohydrates (more than 150 grams a day), you might gain weight. But if you're eating low carbs (under 100 grams a day) and moderate to high fat, you're in the clear. It may take a bit of time to adjust to using fat as fuel, but it will happen.

If you start off eating a lot of fat and taper down to get your calories under control, it can help create a smoother, less fatigued transition into Paleo. Be patient and don't fear the fat! Healthy oils and animal fats, even in excess of 100 grams per day, will actually help you feel better and lose weight, all while curbing cravings. Help yourself to some bacon and eggs smothered in guacamole for breakfast.

## Calorie Deficit

Because you'll be removing such a large part of your diet (vegetable oils, dairy, sugar, and grains make up about 70 percent of the Western diet), you may not fill your plate as high as you normally would. Because most people are overweight in part because they eat too many calories, that can be a really good thing, but don't overdo it.

Eat enough fat, protein, and carbohydrates to keep you satiated, but you shouldn't be starving all the time. In fact, even with less food, people often report feeling less hungry than usual on the Paleolithic diet. Let fullness be your guide. On a scale from 1 to 10, where 1 is so hungry you could faint and 10 is so full you could throw up, try to aim for a 5 to 8 on that scale every time you eat. You should feel comfortably full but not stuffed.

## Frequent Fruity Snacks

While fruit is delicious and nutritious, and it's definitely a part of the Paleolithic diet, don't make all your snacks just fruit. Too much fruit, especially dried fruit, can mess with your blood sugar levels and make you hungry again quickly. Eat some nuts or jerky with that fruit sometimes, or instead of it.

**PALEO COMPASS**

Be sure to stay hydrated on the diet, but remember that fruit juice, with its high glycemic index and low nutrient value, is not on the menu. The same goes for diet sodas made with artificial sweeteners and any other sweetened drinks. Stick with water, or water with a bit of fresh fruit squeezed in it.

## Going Nuts for Nuts

Nuts are often overused on the diet, especially in the beginning when they're the most convenient, portable snack you know of. However, nuts shouldn't be a large part of your daily calories. As far as overall nutrients go, nuts and seeds rank lowest when compared with fruits, vegetables, seafood, lean meats, and even whole grains and milk. And they're the highest calorie foods of all those. Plus, despite their reputation for being high protein, they're no better than grains on an ounce for ounce basis, at around 5 grams per ounce. Opt for leftovers from meals or a *combination* of nuts, fruit, and animal products for snacks. Nuts are a nice addition to the diet, but our ancestors didn't live on them.

## Smoothie Obsession

While smoothies are deliciously sweet and can be nutrient dense, they often lack protein. Depending on a smoothie for breakfast every day can cause blood sugar imbalances. Opt for more protein and fat-dense breakfasts like eggs or leftovers. That will start the day off right and keep you from needing an afternoon siesta. Eat smoothies for breakfast every once in a while or have one as a side to a more substantial breakfast.

# What to Expect in the Beginning

Here's a typical scenario: you've been on the Paleolithic diet for a few days and you're not feeling the *amazing* effects of the diet that so many others before you have. In fact, you feel worse than before you started! Naturally, you're wondering whether the diet really works, and if it's worth it. Almost every Paleo eater has been right where you are. You are not alone and it will get better. Soon.

Because Paleo is much cleaner and less toxic than a normal Western diet, you may experience some (or a lot of) detoxification symptoms, including intense cravings, headaches, and fatigue. Why? You stopped eating some possibly addictive things your body has to work hard to deal with, like gluten, phytic acid, and lectins in grains and legumes; preservatives and other additives; refined oils, flours, and sweeteners; and dairy, which is worse for some people than others.

Because you've probably been eating those things your whole life, your body is going through some serious withdrawal. But it's also *finally* getting a chance to clean out some built up toxins. Without all the harmful foods constantly bombarding your organs and cells, and with the assistance of all the new nutrients from the foods you're now eating, your body is going to take the opportunity to do some much needed cleaning. That purging is exactly what causes the symptoms you may experience. It's like when you do a deep cleaning of your house: you turn it upside down and inside out before it looks immaculate. In the first three days to three weeks of eating Paleo, you may experience:

- Brain fog
- Diarrhea/constipation
- Dizziness
- Fatigue
- Flulike symptoms
- Headaches
- Increased/decreased appetite
- Increased thirst
- Increased urination
- Intense cravings
- Irritability
- Mood swings
- Nausea
- Sinus drainage
- Skin issues

Sounds terrible, right? Don't worry too much: some people don't experience any symptoms at all, and many only experience symptoms for a few days to a week. There's really no way of predicting how long your detoxification period will last, but it's unlikely it will go on for more than a few weeks.

**DAMAGE CONTROL**

If your symptoms become severe, try eating more carbohydrates in the form of sweet potatoes and the other starchy veggies on the diet. Also try eating more fat in the form of fatty meats, extra oils, nuts, and avocados. You may feel awful just from not eating enough food, so upping your portion sizes all around might help. However, if your symptoms don't improve or they get worse, consult a health professional for guidance.

Most people begin to notice at least one thing improve, even in the midst of their detoxification period. They have more energy, but they're really thirsty. Or their skin starts clearing up, but they have slight diarrhea. Maybe they get dull headaches, but they're happily losing weight rapidly at the same time. Your individual detox period will be different from everyone else's.

If you are a coffee or otherwise caffeinated beverage drinker and you're giving that up at the same time, you should almost undoubtedly expect some symptoms. Caffeine is an addictive substance, as you know, and your nervous and endocrine systems will need some time to recover from the withdrawal. You might find that you're a bit grumpy during this time.

Steve, a 55-year-old male, struggled during the first few weeks on the Paleolithic diet. The first day, he needed a nap at 2 P.M. and another at 4 P.M.; he was in bed for the night at 8 P.M. that first night. It got a little easier after a week, and then after two weeks Steve started to feel better. Now when he gets up in the mornings he feels like working out, not guzzling coffee. Steve lost 15 pounds his first month, which was within 5 pounds of his goal!

So when you're wondering whether or not this diet is, in fact, *hurting* you—not helping—remember that after the storm of detoxification subsides, you may very well experience all of the health benefits we've already discussed throughout the book, including weight loss, more energy, healthier skin, and clarity of mind.

We've provided a month's worth of meal plans (see Chapter 18) and grocery lists (see Appendix C) to give you the best chance at success, even if you're feeling like you want to quit. Everything is laid out before you—you just need to shop, cook, and eat the tasty foods you create. Stick with the plan and you will be rewarded!

## The Least You Need to Know

- Your plate should be filled up by about half plant foods and half animal foods.
- Avoid counting calories for weight loss unless you aren't losing weight on the diet after about a month.
- Don't make common beginner missteps like eating too many nuts or having sugary smoothies for breakfast every morning.
- You may experience some discomfort in the first days or weeks of the diet as your body cleans itself out, but it will subside and you'll be delighted you persevered.

# Four-Week Starter Meal Plan

## In This Chapter

- Implementing the four-week meal plan
- Changing the meal plan to fit your life
- Addressing health concerns
- Four weekly menus to start you off right!

Knowledge is power, as we all know, and you now have the power of the Paleolithic diet. It's by far the best choice for humans. But more practical knowledge will empower you further by helping you start the diet and stay on it for good. That's why we've included a four-week meal plan in this chapter. It will teach you what to cook and when, and what you need at the grocery store every week to be prepared.

The meal plan not only tells you what to eat and what to buy, it also helps you save money by not purchasing too much food. You only buy what you need for the week.

## Details of the Meal Plan

The meal plan is a combination of weekly menus, their corresponding grocery shopping lists in Appendix C, and the recipes in Part 3 of this book. It tells you exactly what to eat every day for breakfast, lunch, snack, and dinner, cleverly using leftovers to make it convenient and doable.

The plan is based on our website, paleoplan.com, which is a highly successful meal-planning service for Paleo eaters. The website offers free recipes, original meal plans, and shopping lists every week, and it's helped thousands of people all over the world stay true to the diet. That means the recipes and menus in this book have been tried, tested, and tweaked to fit everyday people's tastes and time constraints. Using the plan, you can make eating Paleo a seamless part of your life. First, though, understanding a few things about it will create a smoother transition.

## Number of People

The meal plan is designed for two people following it together. The shopping list and the recipes themselves provide guidance for what two average people eat. If your household is smaller or larger than two people, you will find information on adjusting the meal plan to fit your needs later in this chapter.

> **PALEO COMPASS**
>
> Because the meal plan is a general guide for two people, use your best judgment when determining how much food each person should get. For instance, if you and your boyfriend are doing the diet together and he is much taller and more active than you, you might consider giving him a slightly larger share of the shared meals. On the other hand, if you are both taller-than-average, active people, you might consider increasing the amount of food you buy and prepare.

## Meals

The four-week meal plan provides three meals and one snack for two people every day. It is made up of relatively simple-to-cook meals that can often be prepared quickly without sacrificing quality. The weekday meals are usually easier to prepare and often consist of recurring items. This is so you can get used to making certain dishes and not have to rely on a recipe every time you enter the kitchen.

The plan takes advantage of weekends to allow for more complex and interesting recipes. You'll often find new and more adventurous recipes on those days. If your workweek isn't Monday through Friday, feel free to adjust the days as necessary.

Some of the meals consist of more than one recipe, in which case a semicolon separates the names of the recipes. If a recipe is found in the book, it is capitalized, as in "Endive Salmon Poppers." If it is a generic food, it will not be capitalized, like "bacon." We also provide you with the chapter in which you can find the recipe.

## Prep Days

We encourage you to take advantage of Sundays as a time to precook and chop items that will be used throughout the week. For instance, if you know the coming Wednesday is a busy day for you, take a look ahead and see what you can do on

Sunday to make Wednesday's meals easier to prepare. Maybe you can chop some veggies or even precook a meal and freeze it. The meal plan includes some suggestions for preparing certain things in advance, but do what makes sense for your schedule.

## Shopping Lists

The shopping lists that correspond to the weekly menus can be found in Appendix C. There's a Staples List that includes things like flour, nuts, oils, and spices, so you can stock up on the nonperishable items you'll need for the month. This makes week-to-week shopping quicker and easier. The weekly Grocery Lists include fresh meat, seafood, eggs, produce, and other items you'll want to buy fresh.

The quantities of some items are left up to you to determine, like "snack serving of fruit." In those cases, you should buy enough fruit for two people for one meal or snack.

## Protein Serving Sizes

In general, each meal is focused around 4 to 6 ounces of meat or fish per serving. The amount of protein in each serving can be found in the nutritional information of each recipe.

**PALEO COMPASS**

*Fruit* or *nuts* or similar terms are often listed in the meal plans without a specific amount. These are generally for snacks. In those cases, it's up to you to decide which types of fruit or nuts you prefer, so you can keep snacks interesting and seasonal based on your location. A good serving size for fruit is 1 medium piece. A decent serving of nuts is an adult-size handful, or about 23 almonds.

## Leftovers

Many of the dinners are designed to provide enough food for leftovers later in the week. When we say leftovers, we mean enough food for a meal for two people. Unless it's explicitly stated, the recipes themselves will make enough for leftovers without modification. When the recipe is good only for two servings, the meal plan will notify you to double the recipe in order to have leftovers. The shopping lists are always appropriate for the amount of food necessary.

## Weekends

While the weekend breakfasts and dinners might be a bit more elaborate, weekend lunches and snacks are opportunities to eat what's left over from the previous week. The meal plan often calls for grazing the fridge and picking out any foods you may have missed over the week. There may be a few pieces of fruit left, some extra chicken, or a salad from the week's lunches. Take this opportunity to finish the week's groceries so you're not throwing anything away, including your hard-earned money.

# Altering the Meal Plan to Fit Your Needs

The meal plan is built for two average people, but not everyone is average or half of a couple. You may live alone or with a lot of people, including kids. You can certainly adjust the meal plan to fit your personal needs, whether that's by changing the amount of food you're preparing or taking special care for health concerns like diabetes or food allergies.

## Going Solo

If you're doing the meal plan on your own, cut the recipes and grocery lists in half. It will just take some simple math when you're at the grocery store and measuring things out in the kitchen.

If you're an athlete or working out regularly while you're doing the meal plan on your own, read Chapter 6 to figure out what adjustments you'll need to make to the menu, if any. It may just mean that you're buying more sweet potatoes and other starchy foods to add to your meals. If you're a very large and very active male athlete doing the meal plan alone, you may be able to keep the serving sizes as they are and eat the whole menu on your own!

**PALEO COMPASS**

All of the recipes found in Part 3 include nutritional information, including calories, and grams of carbs, fat, and protein. So if you're keeping track of any of those numbers this will make it very easy. All the nutritional information was derived from myfitnesspal.com.

## Feeding More Than Two

If you're cooking and shopping for more than two adults, you just need to consider the other eaters' appetites when you're adjusting the recipes and shopping lists. Here are a few examples:

- If you have two small children who, together, eat about as much as one adult, then multiply the shopping lists and recipes by one and a half. That will give you three adult-size servings instead of two every meal.

- If you have three growing teenage boys with colossal appetites, consider multiplying everything by at least three. That would create at least six servings per meal for five people.

> **PALEO COMPASS**
>
> Consider buying things in bulk and maybe even purchasing an extra freezer. That way you can buy and store meat, nuts, seeds, frozen veggies, and frozen fruits in large quantities, making your food budget more manageable.

# Health Concerns

People often ask if they should consult with their doctor before starting this diet. If you feel more comfortable updating your doctor, that's fine. But since this is the way you were physiologically intended to eat, it's not necessary to get your doctor's permission. Unless you have a serious medical issue already, like a genetic inability to digest fats, diabetes, or a severe allergy to certain foods, you should be able to go on the diet freely. We discuss which precautions you should take if you have diabetes or allergies in the following sections. If you have other concerns, consult a nutritionist before starting, preferably one who is knowledgeable about the Paleolithic diet.

## Diabetics

Diabetics often wonder if the Paleolithic diet and meal plan are safe for them. The answer is a resounding yes! As you've learned throughout the book, the diet removes many of the high glycemic foods that cause blood glucose imbalances, which can lead to diabetes. When diabetics start eating Paleo, they usually find that their blood glucose levels decrease dramatically, even in the first few days of being on the diet. There's nothing you need to alter about the diet itself when you're diabetic: you just need to devote some extra care to your blood sugar–lowering medications, if you're on any. If you are on medication or insulin for diabetes, consult your doctor to discuss how you are changing your diet and how he may need to adjust the dose of your medications.

The diet alone will lower your blood sugar levels, so you don't want to lower them too much with pharmaceuticals and cause hypoglycemia. Monitor your blood glucose more closely than usual. Know that if you take too much insulin without eating any high glycemic carbohydrates, your blood sugar may plummet. You may want to experiment with your insulin dosages with your doctor.

## Nut Allergies

With the growing number of food allergies, there's a chance you may not be able to eat one or more of the major ingredients in the diet. If you're sensitive to tree nuts like so many others are, you won't be eating some of the suggested snacks or the recipes using almond flour. In that case, always have jerky and fruit or any other favorite snacks on hand in place of the nut-based snacks in the meal plan. As for the almond flour, a mixture of coconut flour and tapioca flour works well as a substitute. Read Chapter 8 for more information on using coconut flour.

## Egg Allergies

Egg allergies are common, too, and there are things you can do to get around that on the meal plan. Just use meats in the eggs' place in savory dishes. For instance, pan-fry or roast chicken (substitute 2 ounces per egg) and replace it in the omelets. No, it won't be your typical omelet all wrapped up in egg, but it will be a delicious, protein-and-veggie-filled breakfast.

As for the baked goods with eggs, use things like arrowroot (a thickening agent) or flax meal in place of eggs. Here are five good substitutions for one egg:

- 2 tablespoons arrowroot

- 1 teaspoon baking powder plus 1½ tablespoons water plus 1½ tablespoons oil

- 1 tablespoon tapioca plus ¼ cup warm water

- 2 tablespoons applesauce

- "Flax Eggs": Mix 1 tablespoon flax plus 3 tablespoons water. Let sit to gel for 5 minutes. Whisk.

**NUTRITION FACT**

We highly suggest you *not* use most store-bought egg substitutes. Many of them are soy- or corn-based, and some are even made of egg whites! However, there are some more natural egg replacement products that are almost completely Paleo. (Ener-G makes a good one.)

# The Meal Plan

And without further ado, here are the meal plans. Enjoy!

# Week 1

If Sunday is a busy day for you, consider making Sunday's doubled Chicken Fajita Salad lunch recipe and the Paleo Candy Bars on Saturday.

**Sunday**

1. *Breakfast:* Omelet Muffins (recipe in Chapter 9)

2. *Lunch:* Chicken Fajita Salad (recipe in Chapter 11)

3. *Snack:* Paleo Candy Bars (recipe in Chapter 11)

4. *Dinner:* Salmon Cakes with Mango and Cilantro Salsa (recipe in Chapter 13); mixed greens with Simple Salad Dressing (recipe in Chapter 12)

**Monday**

5. *Breakfast:* Eggs with Avocado and Salsa (recipe in Chapter 9)

6. *Lunch:* Leftover Chicken Fajita Salad (recipe in Chapter 11)

7. *Snack:* Leftover Paleo Candy Bars (recipe in Chapter 11)

8. *Dinner:* Easy Pork Loin Chops (recipe in Chapter 14); Fresh Tomatoes with Basil (Chapter 12)

**Tuesday**

9. *Breakfast:* Leftover Omelet Muffins (recipe in Chapter 9)

10. *Lunch:* Leftover Easy Pork Loin Chops (recipe in Chapter 14); mixed greens with Simple Salad Dressing (recipe in Chapter 12)

11. *Snack:* Jerky; fruit

12. *Dinner:* Curry Chicken and Cauliflower Rice (recipe in Chapter 15)

**Wednesday**

13. *Breakfast:* Ham and Applesauce with Almonds (recipe in Chapter 9)

14. *Lunch:* Leftover Curry Chicken and Cauliflower Rice (recipe in Chapter 15)

15. *Snack:* PB & J Paleo Style (recipe in Chapter 11)

16. *Dinner:* Pepper Steak (recipe in Chapter 14)

**Thursday**

17. *Breakfast:* Breakfast Smoothie (recipe in Chapter 10)

18. *Lunch:* Leftover Pepper Steak (recipe in Chapter 14)

19. *Snack:* Jerky; veggies

20. *Dinner:* Cilantro Turkey Burgers (recipe in Chapter 15); Orange, Avocado, and Cashew Salad (recipe in Chapter 11)

**Friday**

21. *Breakfast:* Chorizo Scrambled Eggs (recipe in Chapter 9)

22. *Lunch:* Leftover Cilantro Turkey Burgers (recipe in Chapter 15); mixed greens with Simple Salad Dressing (recipe in Chapter 12)

23. *Snack:* Berries with Balsamic Vinegar and Almonds (recipe in Chapter 11)

24. *Dinner:* Honey-Walnut Chicken (recipe in Chapter 15); Roasted Asparagus (recipe in Chapter 12)

**Saturday**

25. *Breakfast:* Almond Flour Pancakes (recipe in Chapter 10); bacon

26. *Lunch:* Graze leftovers from fridge

27. *Snack:* Graze leftovers from fridge

28. *Dinner:* Paleo Pizza (recipe in Chapter 14)

# Week 2

### Sunday

1. *Breakfast:* Myra's Chopped Mushrooms, Eggs, and Onions (recipe in Chapter 9)

   *Prep: Hard-boil eggs for Monday's lunch.*

2. *Lunch:* Graze leftovers from fridge

3. *Snack:* Graze leftovers from fridge

4. *Dinner:* Baked Sea Bass with Capers and Lemon (recipe in Chapter 13); steamed broccoli with lemon

### Monday

5. *Breakfast:* Leftover Myra's Chopped Mushrooms, Eggs, and Onions (recipe in Chapter 9)

6. *Lunch:* Paleo Niçoise Salad (recipe in Chapter 11)

7. *Snack:* Jerky; fruit

8. *Dinner:* Lime-Cilantro Pork Wraps (recipe in Chapter 14); Salsa Salad (recipe in Chapter 11)

### Tuesday

9. *Breakfast:* Breakfast Smoothie (recipe in Chapter 10)

10. *Lunch:* Leftover Lime-Cilantro Pork Wraps (recipe in Chapter 14)

11. *Snack:* Endive Salmon Poppers (recipe in Chapter 12)

12. *Dinner:* Grilled Chicken Kebabs with Garlic and Cumin (recipe in Chapter 15); Mojo Verde (recipe in Chapter 12); Watermelon with Fresh Herbs (recipe in Chapter 12)

### Wednesday

13. *Breakfast:* Veggies and Eggies (recipe in Chapter 9)

14. *Lunch:* Leftover Grilled Chicken Kebabs with Garlic and Cumin (recipe in Chapter 15); Mojo Verde (recipe in Chapter 12); Watermelon with Fresh Herbs (recipe in Chapter 12)

15. *Snack:* Paleo Trail Mix (recipe in Chapter 11)

16. *Dinner:* Coconut Chicken (recipe in Chapter 15); Chard and Cashew Sauté (recipe in Chapter 12)

### Thursday

17. *Breakfast:* Almost Oatmeal (recipe in Chapter 10); chicken sausage

18. *Lunch:* Leftover Coconut Chicken (recipe in Chapter 15); mixed greens with Simple Salad Dressing (recipe in Chapter 12)

19. *Snack:* Fruit Salad with Cinnamon (recipe in Chapter 11)

20. *Dinner:* Bun-Less Burgers (recipe in Chapter 14); Apple Coleslaw (recipe in Chapter 12)

### Friday

21. *Breakfast:* Sausage Stir-Fry Breakfast (recipe in Chapter 9)

22. *Lunch:* Leftover Bun-Less Burgers (recipe in Chapter 14); leftover Apple Coleslaw (recipe in Chapter 12)

23. *Snack:* Jerky; veggies

24. *Dinner:* Lamb with Sweet Red Peppers (recipe in Chapter 14)

### Saturday

25. *Breakfast:* Western Omelet (recipe in Chapter 9)

26. *Lunch:* Graze leftovers from fridge

27. *Snack:* Graze leftovers from fridge

28. *Dinner:* Grilled Flank Steak with Pineapple Salsa (recipe in Chapter 14)

## Week 3

### Sunday

1. *Breakfast:* Baked Eggs in Bacon Rings (recipe in Chapter 9)

2. *Lunch:* Graze leftovers from fridge

3. *Snack:* Graze leftovers from fridge

4. *Dinner:* Almond Crusted Salmon (recipe in Chapter 13); Sautéed Fennel and Carrots (recipe in Chapter 12)

## Monday

5. *Breakfast:* Fried Eggs with Sweet Potato Hash (recipe in Chapter 9)

6. *Lunch:* Spicy Tuna Salad (recipe in Chapter 11)

7. *Snack:* Jerky; fruit

8. *Dinner:* Grilled Chicken Mediterranean (recipe in Chapter 15); Cantaloupe and Avocado Salad with Honey-Lime Dressing (recipe in Chapter 11)

## Tuesday

9. *Breakfast:* No-Oat "Oatmeal" (recipe in Chapter 10)

10. *Lunch:* Leftover Grilled Chicken Mediterranean (recipe in Chapter 15); leftover Cantaloupe and Avocado Salad with Honey-Lime Dressing (recipe in Chapter 11)

11. *Snack:* Jerky; veggies

12. *Dinner:* Taco Salad (recipe in Chapter 14)

## Wednesday

13. *Breakfast:* Savory Zucchini Fritters (recipe in Chapter 9); sausage links

14. *Lunch:* Leftover Taco Salad (recipe in Chapter 14)

15. *Snack:* Berries with Balsamic Vinegar and Almonds (recipe in Chapter 11)

16. *Dinner:* Turkey Vegetable Meatballs (recipe in Chapter 15); Zucchini and Squash Sauté (recipe in Chapter 12)

## Thursday

17. *Breakfast:* Fruit Salad with Cinnamon (recipe in Chapter 11); bacon (double the recipe for Fruit Salad with Cinnamon)

    *Prep: Hard-boil eggs for Thursday's snack.*

18. *Lunch:* Leftover Turkey Vegetable Meatballs (recipe in Chapter 15); Zucchini and Squash Sauté (recipe in Chapter 12)

19. *Snack:* Guacamole Deviled Eggs (recipe in Chapter 11)

20. *Dinner:* Thai Chicken Wraps (recipe in Chapter 15)

### Friday

21. *Breakfast:* Roasted Pepper and Sausage Omelet (recipe in Chapter 9)

22. *Lunch:* Leftover Thai Chicken Wraps (recipe in Chapter 15)

23. *Snack:* PB & J Paleo Style (recipe in Chapter 11)

24. *Dinner:* Pork Loin with Peppers, Mushrooms, and Onions (recipe in Chapter 14)

### Saturday

25. *Breakfast:* Tapioca Crêpes (recipe in Chapter 10); bacon

26. *Lunch:* Graze leftovers from fridge

27. *Snack:* Graze leftovers from fridge

28. *Dinner:* Osso Buco (recipe in Chapter 14); Spinach Salad (recipe in Chapter 11)

## Week 4

### Sunday

1. *Breakfast:* Carrot Banana Muffins (recipe in Chapter 10)

   *Prep: Hard-boil eggs and cook bacon for Monday's lunch.*

2. *Lunch:* Graze leftovers from fridge

3. *Snack:* Graze leftovers from fridge

4. *Dinner:* Grilled Shrimp and Veggies on a Stick (recipe in Chapter 13)

### Monday

5. *Breakfast:* Shrimp and Avocado Omelet (recipe in Chapter 9)

6. *Lunch:* Chef Salad (recipe in Chapter 11)

7. *Snack:* Leftover Carrot Banana Muffins (recipe in Chapter 10); jerky

8. *Dinner:* Fruited Chicken Thighs (recipe in Chapter 15); mixed greens with Simple Salad Dressing (recipe in Chapter 12)

**Tuesday**

9. *Breakfast:* Leftover Carrot Banana Muffins (recipe in Chapter 10)

10. *Lunch:* Leftover Fruited Chicken Thighs (recipe in Chapter 15); mixed greens with Simple Salad Dressing (recipe in Chapter 12)

11. *Snack:* Jerky; veggies

12. *Dinner:* Salmon with Coconut Cream Sauce (recipe in Chapter 13); Sautéed Fennel and Carrots (recipe in Chapter 12)

**Wednesday**

13. *Breakfast:* Banana Almond Pancakes (recipe in Chapter 10); chicken sausage

14. *Lunch:* Leftover Salmon with Coconut Cream Sauce (recipe in Chapter 13); leftover Sautéed Fennel and Carrots (recipe in Chapter 12)

15. *Snack:* Paleo Candy Bars (recipe in Chapter 11)

16. *Dinner:* Beef Pot Roast (recipe in Chapter 14); Roasted Beets with Balsamic Glaze (recipe in Chapter 12)

**Thursday**

17. *Breakfast:* Breakfast Smoothie (recipe in Chapter 10)

18. *Lunch:* Leftover Beef Pot Roast (recipe in Chapter 14); leftover Roasted Beets with Balsamic Glaze (recipe in Chapter 12)

19. *Snack*: PB & J Paleo Style (recipe in Chapter 11)

20. *Dinner:* Chicken and Sweet Potatoes with Shallots (recipe in Chapter 15)

**Friday**

21. *Breakfast:* Scrambled Eggs with Bacon and Vegetables (recipe in Chapter 9)

22. *Lunch:* Leftover Chicken and Sweet Potatoes with Shallots (recipe in Chapter 15)

23. *Snack:* Jerky; fruit

24. *Dinner:* Gingery Broccoli and Beef (recipe in Chapter 14)

**Saturday**

25. *Breakfast:* Summer Vegetable Frittata (recipe in Chapter 9)

26. *Lunch:* Graze leftovers from fridge

27. *Snack:* Graze leftovers from fridge

28. *Dinner:* Coconut Lamb with Cauliflower "Rice" (recipe in Chapter 14)

## The Least You Need to Know

- Following the four-week meal plan is simple when you know a few details about it.
- Whether you're single or trying to feed a family, you can easily alter the meal plan to fit your needs.
- Unless you have health concerns, you should be able to start the diet without your doctor's supervision.
- Follow the weekly menus for a month and you won't even have to think about whether foods are Paleo or not.

**antinutrient**   A natural or synthetic compound that interferes with the absorption of nutrients. Examples include the phytic acid and enzyme inhibitors in grains and the tannins in wine.

**carbohydrates**   One of the three macronutrients that provide calories, the others being protein and fat. They can be simple sugars like glucose and fructose or more complex like starch and fiber. Carbohydrates are found in abundance in grains, refined sugars, legumes, vegetables, and fruits. Your body uses carbohydrates as energy for your muscles and organs, although it can also use fat and protein. *See also* fat; protein.

**carcinogen**   Any substance that is capable of causing cancer.

**cold-pressed virgin** and **extra-virgin oils**   Oils that have this designation are not heated at high temperatures, chemically deodorized, bleached, or chemically treated in any way to refine them. They are produced during the first mechanical pressing of the seed or fruit.

**cortisol**   A hormone produced and secreted by the adrenal glands in response to low blood sugar or other stressful situations. Its main purpose is to tell the liver and muscles to secrete glucose into the bloodstream.

**fat**   One of the three macronutrients that provides calories in our diet. There are many kinds of fats, including saturated, monounsaturated, and polyunsaturated. All oils and fats are a combination of saturated, monounsaturated, and polyunsaturated fatty acids. Fat is found in abundance in certain meats, dairy, nuts, and seeds. Every cell in your body requires fat, and it's very important for proper nerve function, hormone balance, and vitamin absorption. Fatty acids are also the preferred fuel for the heart and skeletal muscles. *See also* carbohydrates; fatty acids; monounsaturated fatty acids; polyunsaturated fatty acids; omega-3 fatty acids; omega-6 fatty acids; protein; saturated fatty acids.

**fatty acids**   Fatty acids are the building blocks of fats and oils. They are constructed of a carboxylic acid with a long "tail" made mostly of carbon atoms. The long tails are either saturated by hydrogen, meaning they don't contain any double bonds, or they are unsaturated, meaning they contain one or more double bonds. All fatty acids are named according to the number of double bonds they contain.

**food sensitivities**   A negative immune response to a certain food.

**glucose**   A type of carbohydrate that is a simple sugar, made of carbon, oxygen, and hydrogen. It's an important energy source in living organisms, and it's a building block for many other carbohydrates.

**high-density lipoprotein (HDL)**   Referred to as "good" cholesterol, a combination of protein, triglycerides, and cholesterol that transports cholesterol from cells of the body back to the liver.

**lactose intolerant**   The term for someone who lacks the enzyme lactase to digest the sugar, lactose, in milk.

**legume**   A plant in the family *Fabaceae*, including pinto and black beans, lentils, soy, and peanuts.

**low-density lipoprotein (LDL)**   Referred to as "bad" cholesterol, a combination of protein, triglycerides, and cholesterol that transports cholesterol from the liver to other cells of the body for use.

**macronutrient**   Any one of the three classes of chemical compounds we consume in the largest quantities, and from which we derive calories from—carbohydrates, fats, and proteins.

**monounsaturated fatty acids**   These have one double bond in their structure, hence the *mono*. They are more susceptible to damage by heat, light, and oxygen than saturated fatty acids. They are found in foods like olive oil, lard, and other animal fats. They're considered to be heart-healthy fats, even by conventional standards.

**omega-3 fatty acids**   Polyunsaturated fatty acids found in cold-water fish such as salmon and mackerel, certain nuts and seeds, and, in lesser amounts, leafy green vegetables. One of the double bonds is located on the third carbon atom from the end of the carbon chain, which is why it's called omega-*3*. These fatty acids are necessary to humans and they are anti-inflammatory.

**omega-6 fatty acids**   Polyunsaturated fatty acids found abundantly in nuts and seeds. One of the double bonds is located on the sixth carbon atom from the end of the carbon chain, which is why it's called omega-*6*. These fatty acids are also necessary to humans, but they are inflammatory.

**oxidized**   The state of an oil or fat after it is exposed to too much heat, light, and air. The less stable the fatty acids are, the more easily they oxidize.

**Paleo**   A shortened version of the term *Paleolithic diet* to refer to that diet or the lifestyle that accompanies it.

**Paleolithic diet**   A term for the diet that mimics the diet of humans' Paleolithic ancestors, which omits grains, beans, refined sugar, dairy, and most seed oils, and includes meat, fish, eggs, fruit, vegetables, and some nuts and seeds.

**pastured**   Refers to animals that have been raised almost completely or entirely on a pasture, eating the foods they were designed to eat. The quality of the fats in those animals is much more in line with what our ancestors would have gotten from the wild animals they ate.

**polyunsaturated fatty acids**   Fatty acids that have more than one double bond in their structure, hence the word *poly*. Omega-3s and omega-6s are polyunsaturated.

**protein**   One of the three macronutrients that provide us with calories, along with fat and carbohydrates. It is composed of amino acids, which are made of nitrogen, carbon, and oxygen. High-protein foods are meat and organs, fish, eggs, dairy, and nuts, usually in that order. You need protein for muscle and bone growth, hormone production, and to repair and heal damaged tissue, among many other functions. *See also* carbohydrates; fat.

**saturated fatty acids**   Fatty acids whose carbon chain is completely saturated by hydrogen and cannot absorb any more hydrogen atoms. Saturated fat is generally solid at room temperature, and it's found in abundance in animal fats and tropical oils like coconut and palm.

**trans fats**   Type of fats made by hydrogenating, or adding hydrogen molecules, to unsaturated fats. The process unnaturally turns unsaturated fats or oils into saturated fats in order to make them solid at room temperature and to have a longer shelf life. It changes the structure into something unrecognizable by the body. They're found in many processed foods, especially fast food, cookies, and other prepackaged baked goods. They're now known to contribute to heart disease.

**unsaturated fatty acids**   Fatty acids, like monounsaturated fatty acids and polyunsaturated fatty acids (omega-3 and omega-6), whose carbon tails are not saturated by hydrogen. They have one or more double bonds.

# Resources

## Books

Cordain, Loren, PhD. *The Paleo Diet (Revised Edition).* John Wiley & Sons, 2011.

Cordain, Loren, PhD, and Joe Friel, MS. *The Paleo Diet for Athletes.* Rodale, 2005.

De Vany, Arthur. *The New Evolution Diet.* Rodale, 2011.

Eades, Michael R., MD, and Mary Dan Eades, MD. *Protein Power.* Bantam, 1999.

Fallon, Sally, and Mary Enig. *Nourishing Traditions.* New Trends Publishing, 1999.

Price, Weston A., DDS. *Nutrition and Physical Degeneration.* Price-Pottinger Nutrition Foundation, 2000.

Sisson, Mark. *The Primal Blueprint.* Primal Nutrition, Inc., 2009.

Stevenson, Nell, and Loren Cordain. *The Paleo Diet Cookbook.* John Wiley & Sons, 2010.

Taubes, Gary. *Good Calories, Bad Calories.* Anchorbooks, 2008.

Wolf, Rob. *The Paleo Solution.* Victory Belt Publishing, 2010.

## Online Resources

### Athletes

Dr. Mauro Di Pasquale (Sports Medicine physician, former world-class athlete): metabolicdiet.com

Nell Stephenson (IronMan athlete and Paleo nutritionist): nellstephenson.com

## Blogs and Podcasts

Chris Kresser, L.Ac: chriskresser.com

Chris Masterjohn: blog.cholesterol-and-health.com

Denise Minger: rawfoodsos.com

Everyday Paleo: everydaypaleo.com

Free The Animal: freetheanimal.com

Hunt.Gather.Love: huntgatherlove.com

Livin' La Vida Low Carb: livinlavidalowcarb.com

Loren Cordain: thepaleodiet.blogspot.com

Marks Daily Apple: marksdailyapple.com

Michael R. Eades, MD: proteinpower.com/drmike

Paleo Plan: paleoplan.com/blog

Robb Wolf: robbwolf.com

The Weston A. Price Foundation: westonaprice.org/blogs

Whole Health Source: wholehealthsource.com

## Family Resources

Everyday Paleo: everydaypaleo.com

## Fish and Seafood Safety Guides

Monterey Bay Aquarium: montereybayaquarium.org/cr/seafoodwatch.aspx

National Resources Defense Council: nrdc.org/health/effects/mercury/guide.asp

## Food Allergies and Sensitivities

Ener-G (egg replacement for people with allergies): ener-g.com/egg-replacer.html

Food sensitivities testing: paleoplan.com/private-paleo-coaching/; enterolab.com

## Free Online Diet and Weight Loss Journals

FitDay: fitday.com

My Fitness Pal: myfitnesspal.com

NutritionData: nutritiondata.com

## Kitchen

Green Pan: green-pan.com

Vitamix Blender: vitamix.com

## Meal-Planning Service

Paleo Plan: paleoplan.com

## Ordering or Sourcing Foods

Almond flour: coconutsecret.com

Almond or other nut butters: futtersnutbutters.com

Coconut products (aminos—tastes like soy sauce, flour, nectar, and oil): coconutsecret.com

Eggs: localharvest.org

Granola: paleopeople.com

Honey: localharvest.org

Meat: eatwild.com; eatwellguide.org; grasslandbeef.com; grassfedtraditions.com

Nuts: nutsonline.com

Produce: doortodoororganics.com; localharvest.com

Raw milk: realmilk.com/where.html

Seafood: wildpacificsalmon.com

## Prepackaged Meals and Snacks

Caveman Cookies: cavemancookies.com

Paleo Brands: paleobrands.com

Paleo Kits: stevesoriginal.com

Paleo People: paleopeople.com

Paleo Treats: paleotreats.com

Primal Pacs: primalpacs.com

Slant Shack Jerky: slantshackjerky.com

Tanka Bars: tankabar.com

U.S. Wellness Meats: grasslandbeef.com

You Bars: youbars.com

# Meal Plan Grocery Shopping Lists

Eating Paleo is a big shift from what most Americans do, and that's a positive thing! It involves planning, cooking, and regular shopping trips, instead of buying prepackaged foods that can be stored almost indefinitely. You have to buy fresh produce weekly, as well as meat if you don't buy it in bulk. This shift in priorities—avoiding processed, packaged, "convenience" foods—comes with the reward of feeling better, having more energy, and getting leaner.

Use the following lists with the meal plan laid out in Chapter 18. The Staples List includes basic items you'll need for the entire month, like flours, nuts, and spices. Buy everything on that list in the first week and you'll have all the staples you need for the month.

The weekly Grocery Lists contain things you'll need to buy fresh every week, such as meat, seafood, eggs, vegetables, and fruit. The lists can be torn out of the book and brought to the grocery store every week. Use the check boxes beside the items to keep track of what you've bought. Before you go shopping, check off what you already have in your house, so you don't buy too much food. For instance, if the list says you need eight eggs for the week and you still have four eggs left over from the week before, you'll only need to buy a half dozen instead of a dozen for the upcoming week. That way, you'll just have a few left over for weekend meals when we suggest you "graze the fridge for leftovers." Also, if the grocery list calls for only four slices of bacon or three stalks of celery for the week, go ahead and buy a small package of bacon or an entire bunch of celery. You'll have an opportunity to use those left overs throughout the week. Saving money is a big priority of this meal plan, so feel confident that you'll eat everything you buy.

We highly encourage you to buy foods that are as natural as possible. Look for labels that say organic, grass-fed, pasture-raised, and nitrate and nitrite free.

# 30-Day Staples List

You'll need the following (generally nonperishable) items for the whole month. If you don't already have them on hand, buy them along with the Week 1 Grocery List.

- ❏ Almond flour, 1¼ lb.
- ❏ Almonds, sliced or slivered, 1 lb.
- ❏ Almonds, whole, 1 lb.
- ❏ Aluminum foil
- ❏ Apple cider vinegar, 16 fl. oz.
- ❏ Applesauce, unsweetened organic, 47-oz. jar
- ❏ Baking soda
- ❏ Balsamic vinegar, 17 fl. oz.
- ❏ Basil
- ❏ Bay leaves
- ❏ Black pepper
- ❏ Caraway seeds
- ❏ Cardamom
- ❏ Cashews, whole, 8 oz.
- ❏ Cayenne
- ❏ Celery seed
- ❏ Chili powder
- ❏ Chives
- ❏ Chunky almond butter, 20-oz. jar
- ❏ Coconut aminos, 8 fl. oz.
- ❏ Coconut flour, 3 oz.
- ❏ Coconut oil, 12 fl. oz.
- ❏ Curry powder
- ❏ Dijon mustard, 9½ oz.
- ❏ Dill weed (optional, may use fresh dill)
- ❏ Dried blueberries, 3 oz.
- ❏ Dried currants, 3 oz.
- ❏ Dried pitted dates, 3 oz.

- ❏ Extra-virgin olive oil, 500 mL
- ❏ Fennel seed
- ❏ Flaxseeds (keep refrigerated and grind right before use), 4 oz.
- ❏ Frozen mixed berries, 2 lb.
- ❏ Garlic powder
- ❏ Garlic salt (granulated garlic)
- ❏ Golden raisins, 4 oz.
- ❏ Grade B pure maple syrup, 8 fl. oz.
- ❏ Ground almonds or hazelnuts, 4 oz.
- ❏ Ground chipotle
- ❏ Ground cinnamon
- ❏ Ground cloves
- ❏ Ground coriander
- ❏ Ground cumin
- ❏ Ground ginger
- ❏ Honey, raw, 12 oz.
- ❏ Hot pepper sauce, $2\frac{1}{2}$ to 5 fl. oz.
- ❏ Italian seasoning blend
- ❏ Jerky, 4 lb.
- ❏ Lemon juice, 8 fl. oz.
- ❏ Lime juice, $2\frac{1}{2}$ fl. oz.
- ❏ Muffin paper liners
- ❏ Nutmeg, whole
- ❏ Oregano
- ❏ Paprika
- ❏ Parchment paper
- ❏ Pumpkin seeds, 4 oz.
- ❏ Red chili flakes
- ❏ Rosemary (optional)
- ❏ Sage
- ❏ Sea salt

❑ Sesame oil, 5 fl. oz.

❑ Shredded coconut, unsweetened, 1½ lb.

❑ Sunflower seeds, raw, 4 oz.

❑ Tapioca flour (tapioca starch), 5 oz.

❑ Tarragon

❑ Thyme

❑ Walnuts, chopped, 12 oz.

❑ Walnuts or pecans, 1 lb.

❑ White pepper

❑ Wooden skewers

# Week 1 Grocery List

## Meat and Seafood

❑ Bacon, 4 strips

❑ Boneless, skinless chicken breasts, 2 lb.

❑ Boneless, skinless chicken breasts, 4 (5 oz. each)

❑ Boneless pork loin chops, 4 (5 oz. each)

❑ Ground turkey, 1 lb.

❑ Ham (Applegate recommended), 1¾ lb.

❑ Hard chorizo (with no filler ingredients), ¼ lb.

❑ Italian sausage, 1 large

❑ Round steak, about ½ in. thick, 1 lb.

❑ Salmon fillet (skinned, with bones removed), 1 lb.

## Vegetables and Fresh Herbs

❑ Asparagus, 1 large bunch (about 20 spears)

❑ Carrots, 4 large

❑ Cauliflower, 1 head

❑ Cherry or grape tomatoes, 2 pints

❑ Cucumber, 1 (6-in.)

❏ Diced fresh vegetables of choice for Omelet Muffins (an extra onion, bell pepper, and small head of broccoli or bunch of asparagus recommended), 4 cups

❏ Fresh basil, 1 package/bunch

❏ Fresh cilantro, 2 bunches

❏ Fresh ginger root, 1 (2-in.)

❏ Fresh thyme, 1 package/bunch

❏ Garlic, 6 cloves

❏ Green bell peppers, 3 (if using green bell peppers where substitution suggested, buy 2 red and 3 green)

❏ Green onions, 1 small bunch

❏ Jalapeño pepper, 1

❏ Mixed greens, 4 handfuls

❏ Red bell peppers, 2

❏ Red leaf or romaine lettuce, 2 large heads

❏ Red onion, 1 large

❏ Spinach, arugula (rocket), or watercress, 3 handfuls

❏ Tomatoes, 4 medium

❏ Veggies of choice, snack serving

❏ White button or cremini mushrooms, 10 medium

❏ Yellow onions, 4

❏ Zucchini, 1 (10- to 12-in.)

## Fruit

❏ Avocados, 4

❏ Berries of choice, 2 pints

❏ Fruit of choice, snack serving

❏ Mango, 1 large

❏ Orange, 1 large

## Other

- ❏ Canned unsweetened coconut milk, 1 (13.6-fl.-oz.) can
- ❏ Carob powder or cocoa (optional), ¼ cup
- ❏ Eggs, 32
- ❏ Marinara, with no added sugar, 1 (8-fl.-oz.) can or jar
- ❏ Salsa, 1 (4-oz.) jar
- ❏ Soda water (optional), 1 (10-fl.-oz.) can or bottle
- ❏ Unsweetened almond milk, 8 fl. oz.

# Week 2 Grocery List

## Meat and Seafood

- ❏ Bacon, 12 strips
- ❏ Beef flank steak, 1 lb.
- ❏ Boneless, skinless chicken breasts, 2 lb.
- ❏ Boneless leg of lamb, 1 lb.
- ❏ Chicken sausage, 8 oz.
- ❏ Ground beef or turkey, lean, 1 lb.
- ❏ Ham, ¼ lb.
- ❏ Pork tenderloin, 1 lb.
- ❏ Sausage, ½ lb.
- ❏ Sea bass fillets (or any firm white fish), 1 lb.
- ❏ Smoked salmon, 4 oz.

## Vegetables

- ❏ Broccoli, 1 lb.
- ❏ Butter lettuce, 2 heads
- ❏ Celery stalk, 1 large
- ❏ Cherry tomatoes, 1 pint
- ❏ Endive, 1 to 2 heads
- ❏ Fresh cilantro, 3 bunches

❑ Fresh dill, 2 sprigs (dried may also be used)

❑ Fresh herbs of choice (a few sprigs of mint, cilantro, parsley, and/or basil recommended), handful

❑ Fresh parsley, 1 bunch

❑ Garlic, 7 cloves

❑ Green beans, 12 large

❑ Green bell peppers, 2

❑ Green chili pepper, 1 small

❑ Jalapeño pepper, 1 small

❑ Kale, 4 leaves

❑ Mixed greens, 4 handfuls

❑ Red bell peppers, 5 large

❑ Red onions, 2

❑ Red or green cabbage, 1 small head

❑ Roma tomatoes, 4

❑ Spinach, 6 handfuls (1 handful optional)

❑ Swiss chard, 1 large bunch

❑ Tomatoes, 2 medium

❑ Veggies of choice, snack serving

❑ White button mushrooms, 12 medium

❑ Yellow onions, 3

## Fruit

❑ Apple, sweet (such as Honeycrisp, Golden Delicious, or Fuji), 1

❑ Apple, tart (such as Granny Smith or Braeburn), 1

❑ Avocados, 3

❑ Fresh pineapple, 4 slices (or canned rings in juice)

❑ Fruit of choice, snack serving

❑ Lemons, 4

❑ Lime, 1

❑ Orange, 1

❑ Watermelon, ¼ large

## Other

❏ Canned tuna (oil-packed albacore suggested), 2 (6-oz.) cans

❏ Canned unsweetened coconut milk, 6 fl. oz.

❏ Capers, 1 (3.5-oz.) jar

❏ Chicken broth, 4 fl. oz.

❏ Eggs, 2 dozen

❏ Kalamata olives, pitted, ½ cup

❏ Unsweetened almond milk, 8 fl. oz.

❏ Whole dulse leaf, 1 oz.

# Week 3 Grocery List

## Meat and Seafood

❏ Bacon, 10 strips

❏ Boneless, skinless chicken breasts, 4 (5 oz. each)

❏ Boneless, skinless chicken breasts, 1 lb.

❏ Ground beef or turkey, lean, 1 lb.

❏ Ground turkey, 1 lb.

❏ Pork loin, 1 lb.

❏ Salmon fillets, 1 lb.

❏ Sausage, 10 links

❏ Smoked beef, 4 thin slices

❏ Veal shanks, 4 (or 1 small veal roast)

## Vegetables

❏ Bibb or romaine lettuce, 1 large head

❏ Broccoli, 1 small head

❏ Butter lettuce, 1 head (or 4 handfuls mixed greens, optional)

❏ Carrots, 9 medium

❏ Celery stalk, 1

❏ Cherry or grape tomatoes, 1 pint

❑ Fennel bulbs, 2

❑ Fresh cilantro, 1 bunch

❑ Fresh parsley, 1 small bunch

❑ Garlic, 9 cloves

❑ Green bell peppers, 2

❑ Green onions, 1 large bunch (9 stalks needed)

❑ Jalapeño pepper, 1

❑ Napa cabbage, 1 small

❑ Poblano pepper, 1

❑ Porcini mushrooms, 3

❑ Red bell peppers, 2

❑ Red onion, 1

❑ Romaine hearts, 1 bag of 3

❑ Spinach, 1 bunch

❑ Sweet potato or yam, 1 medium

❑ Tomatoes, 2 medium

❑ Veggies of choice, snack serving

❑ White button mushrooms, 9

❑ Yellow onions, 4

❑ Yellow summer squash, 2 (6- to 8-in.)

## Fruit

❑ Apples, 2

❑ Avocados, 4

❑ Banana, 1

❑ Berries of choice, 2 pints

❑ Blueberries, 1 pint

❑ Cantaloupe, 1

❑ Fruit of choice, snack serving

❑ Lemons, 6

❑ Limes, 2

❑ Oranges, 2

## Other

- ❑ Black olives, sliced, 1 (6-oz.) can
- ❑ Canned tuna (oil-packed albacore recommended), 2 (6-oz.) cans
- ❑ Canned unsweetened coconut milk, 1 (13.6-fl.-oz.) can
- ❑ Capers, 1 (3.5-oz.) jar
- ❑ Chicken broth, 3 fl. oz.
- ❑ Diced tomatoes, 1 (14.5-oz.) can
- ❑ Eggs, 2 dozen
- ❑ Green olives, pitted, 20
- ❑ Kalamata olives, pitted, 16 to 18 large
- ❑ Salsa, 1 (8-oz.) jar
- ❑ Tomato sauce, 1 (6-oz.) can
- ❑ Unsweetened almond milk, 2 fl. oz.

# Week 4 Grocery List

## Meat and Seafood

- ❑ Bacon, 6 strips
- ❑ Beef pot roast, rump roast, or chuck shoulder, lean, 2 to 3 lb.
- ❑ Boneless, skinless chicken breasts, 4 (5 oz. each)
- ❑ Chicken sausage, 8 oz.
- ❑ Chicken thighs (skin on), 4 (6 oz. each)
- ❑ Ham (boneless, skinless chicken breasts may be substituted), ½ lb.
- ❑ Lamb fillet (tenderloin or steak), 1 lb.
- ❑ Petite sirloin beef steak, 1 lb.
- ❑ Salmon fillet, 1¾ lb.
- ❑ Shrimp, peeled and deveined, 1 lb.

## Vegetables

- ❑ Beets, 5 or 6 (about 3- to 4-in.)
- ❑ Broccoli, 1 lb.
- ❑ Carrots, 13
- ❑ Cauliflower, 1 head
- ❑ Celery stalks, 5
- ❑ Cherry tomatoes, 1 pint
- ❑ Fennel bulbs, 2
- ❑ Fresh basil, 1 package (several sprigs)
- ❑ Fresh cilantro, 1 small bunch
- ❑ Fresh rosemary, 1 sprig
- ❑ Fresh thyme, 1 sprig
- ❑ Garlic, 17 cloves
- ❑ Ginger root, 1 (2-in.)
- ❑ Green bell pepper, 1
- ❑ Green onions, 1 small bunch (5 stalks needed)
- ❑ Mixed greens, 4 handfuls
- ❑ Red bell peppers, 2
- ❑ Red leaf lettuce, 1 head
- ❑ Red onions, 2
- ❑ Shallots, 6 large
- ❑ Snack serving, veggies of choice
- ❑ Spinach, 2 handfuls
- ❑ Sweet potatoes, 4 medium
- ❑ Tomatoes, 7 medium
- ❑ Yellow onions, 4
- ❑ Yellow summer squash, 1 (6- to 8-in.)
- ❑ Zucchini, 5 (6- to 8-in.)

## Fruit

❑ Apples, 2 medium

❑ Avocados, 2

❑ Bananas, 7

❑ Berries of choice, 1 pint

❑ Blueberries, 1 pint

❑ Fruit of choice, snack serving

❑ Lemons, 3

❑ Lime, 1

❑ Orange, 1 (zest only needed)

## Other

❑ Almond milk, 8 fl. oz.

❑ Canned unsweetened coconut milk, 3 (13.6-fl.-oz.) cans

❑ Carob powder or cocoa (optional), ¼ cup

❑ Chicken broth, 8 fl. oz.

❑ Eggs, 29

# Energy and Macronutrient Levels of Foods

The following table contains some common foods with their macronutrient, or carbohydrate, protein, and fat concentrations. For more information on these or other foods' nutritional content, go to nutritiondata.com.

| | Calories | Protein (g) | Carbohydrates (g) | Fat (g) |
|---|---|---|---|---|
| **Almonds** 1 oz. (23 almonds) | 163 | 6 | 6.1 | 14 |
| **Apple** 2¾-in. diameter, raw with peel | 77 | 0.4 | 21 | 0.3 |
| **Asparagus** 4 spears, fresh, raw | 13 | 1.4 | 2.5 | 0.1 |
| **Avocado** ¼ fruit | 80 | 1 | 4.3 | 7.4 |
| **Bacon** 1 slice, cooked | 43 | 3 | 0.1 | 3.3 |
| **Bagel** 1 4-in. bagel, plain | 285 | 11 | 56.5 | 1.7 |
| **Banana** 1 medium | 105 | 1.3 | 27 | 0.4 |
| **Beef, ground** 4 oz., 95% lean, pan-broiled | 193 | 29.7 | 0 | 7.4 |
| **Black beans** ½ cup, canned | 114 | 7.6 | 20.4 | 0.5 |
| **Blueberries** ½ cup, fresh | 42 | 0.6 | 10.7 | 0.2 |
| **Bologna** 1 slice | 87 | 2.9 | 1.1 | 7.9 |

*continues*

*continued*

| | Calories | Protein (g) | Carbohydrates (g) | Fat (g) |
|---|---|---|---|---|
| **Bread, whole wheat**<br>1 slice | 66 | 2.7 | 11.9 | 0.9 |
| **Broccoli**<br>½ cup, fresh, raw | 15 | 1.3 | 3 | 0.2 |
| **Brownie**<br>1 2-in. square | 243 | 2.7 | 39 | 10 |
| **Burger King hamburger**<br>1 sandwich | 333 | 17 | 32.8 | 14.7 |
| **Butter**<br>1 TB., regular, unsalted | 102 | 0.1 | 0 | 11.5 |
| **Cantaloupe**<br>½ cup, fresh | 30 | 0.7 | 7.2 | 0.2 |
| **Carrot**<br>1 medium, fresh, raw | 25 | 0.6 | 5.8 | 0.2 |
| **Cashews**<br>1 oz. | 157 | 5.2 | 8.6 | 12.4 |
| **Cheese, American**<br>1 oz. | 106 | 6.3 | 0.5 | 9 |
| **Chicken**<br>3.5 oz., broiled, light meat | 173 | 30.9 | 0 | 4.5 |
| **Coconut milk**<br>½ cup, canned | 223 | 2.3 | 3.2 | 24.1 |
| **Corn**<br>½ cup, frozen | 66 | 2.3 | 16 | 0.4 |
| **Egg**<br>1 large, hard-boiled | 78 | 6.3 | 0.6 | 5.3 |
| **Grapes**<br>10 medium, with skin | 16 | 0.2 | 4.1 | 0.1 |
| **Green beans**<br>½ cup, fresh, boiled | 22 | 1.2 | 4.9 | 0.2 |
| **Lettuce, romaine**<br>1 cup, shredded | 8 | 0.6 | 1.6 | 0.1 |
| **McDonald's Big Mac**<br>1 sandwich | 563 | 25.9 | 44 | 32.8 |
| **Milk**<br>1 cup, 2% fat | 122 | 8 | 11.7 | 4.8 |

|  | Calories | Protein (g) | Carbohydrates (g) | Fat (g) |
|---|---|---|---|---|
| **Mushrooms** | | | | |
| ½ cup, white, fresh, raw | 8 | 1 | 1.1 | 0.1 |
| **Olive oil** | | | | |
| 1 TB. | 119 | 0 | 0 | 13.5 |
| **Onion** | | | | |
| ½ cup, fresh, raw | 32 | 0.9 | 7.5 | 0.08 |
| **Orange** | | | | |
| 2⅝-in. diameter, fresh | 65 | 1 | 16.3 | 0.3 |
| **Pasta** | | | | |
| 1 cup, spaghetti, cooked | 221 | 8.1 | 43.2 | 1.3 |
| **Peach** | | | | |
| 2½-in. diameter, fresh | 51 | 1.2 | 12.4 | 0.3 |
| **Peanut butter** | | | | |
| 2 TB., smooth | 188 | 8 | 6.3 | 16 |
| **Peas, sweet** | | | | |
| ½ cup, fresh, boiled | 62 | 4.1 | 11.4 | 0.2 |
| **Pepper, green or red** | | | | |
| ½ cup, fresh, raw | 15 | 0.6 | 3.5 | 0.1 |
| **Pork loin** | | | | |
| 4 oz., broiled | 274 | 31 | 0 | 15.7 |
| **Potato** | | | | |
| 1 medium, baked in skin | 161 | 4.3 | 36.6 | 0.2 |
| **Raisins** | | | | |
| ½ cup packed, seedless | 247 | 2.5 | 65 | 0.4 |
| **Rice, white** | | | | |
| ½ cup, boiled | 100 | 2 | 22.4 | 0.2 |
| **Salmon** | | | | |
| 4 oz., Atlantic, wild, cooked | 206 | 28.8 | 0 | 9.1 |
| **Shrimp** | | | | |
| 4 large, fresh, steamed | 26 | 5 | 0.3 | 0.4 |
| **Strawberries** | | | | |
| ½ cup, halves, fresh | 24 | 0.5 | 5.8 | 0.2 |
| **Tomato** | | | | |
| ½ cup, fresh, raw | 16 | 0.8 | 3.5 | 0.2 |
| **Tuna (canned)** | | | | |
| 3 oz., light, in water | 99 | 21.7 | 0 | 0.7 |

*continues*

*continued*

|  | Calories | Protein (g) | Carbohydrates (g) | Fat (g) |
|---|---|---|---|---|
| **Turkey** |  |  |  |  |
| 4 oz., roasted, light meat only | 176 | 34 | 0 | 3.3 |
| **Watermelon** |  |  |  |  |
| ½ cup, fresh | 23 | 0.5 | 5.8 | 0.1 |

*All information from the USDA National Nutrient Database for Standard Reference*

# Nutrient Comparison: Western Diet vs. Paleo

The following is a comparison of the nutrient levels of a typical Western diet and the Paleolithic diet. The 1-day diets are both around 2,000 calories. The nutrients compared are important vitamins and minerals, ratios of fatty acids, and the amounts of each of the three macronutrients (carbohydrates, proteins, and fats), fiber, and sugar. The "%DV" is the percentage of the recommended daily value of a nutrient as set forth by the Food and Drug Administration (FDA). All of those recommended daily values are based on a 2,000-calorie diet.

## Typical Paleolithic Diet

### Breakfast

- Roasted Pepper and Sausage Omelet (recipe in Chapter 9)
- ½ cup sautéed sweet potatoes

### Lunch

- 4 oz. Cilantro Turkey Burger (recipe in Chapter 15) with ½ avocado
- 2 cups raw spinach
- 1 cup cantaloupe

### Snack

- 2 oz. beef jerky
- 10 strawberries
- ½ cup blueberries

### Dinner

- 4 oz. baked salmon
- 1 cup Cauliflower Rice (recipe in Chapter 12)
- 1½ cups steamed broccoli

### Dessert

- Carrot Banana Muffin (recipe in Chapter 10)

# Typical Western Diet

### Breakfast

- 1 cup Cheerios with ¾ cup skim milk
- 2 cups coffee with cream and sugar

### Snack

- Potato chips (about 25 chips)

### Lunch

- McDonald's cheeseburger and small fries
- 12 oz. Coke

### Snack

- Granola bar

### Dinner

- 1 cup spaghetti with ¾ cup marinara sauce
- 3 oz. chicken

### Dessert

- ½ cup chocolate ice cream

| Nutrient | Paleo | %Calories | Western | %Calories |
|---|---|---|---|---|
| Calories | 1,958 | | 1,952 | |
| Carbohydrates | 119 g | 24% | 274 g | 56% |
| Fiber (25 g recommended by FDA) | 42 g | | 19 g | |
| Sugar | 67 g | | 89 g | |
| Glycemic load (target is 100/day or less) | 47 | | 129 | |
| Fat | 109 g | 50% | 63 g | 29% |
| Cholesterol | 593 mg | | 134 mg | |
| Protein | 133 g | 27% | 76 g | 16% |
| *Vitamins* | | *%DV* | | *%DV* |
| Vitamin A | 48,876 IU | 978% | 3,272 IU | 65% |
| Vitamin C | 597 mg | 995% | 37 mg | 62% |
| Vitamin D | 30 IU | 8% | 111 IU | 28% |
| Vitamin E | 27 mg | 135% | 5.7 mg | 28% |
| Vitamin K | 1,610 mcg | 2012% | 35.1 mcg | 44% |
| Thiamin (Vit $B_1$) | 1.5 mg | 103% | 1.3 mg | 90% |
| Riboflavin (Vit $B_2$) | 2.6 mg | 150% | 1.5 mg | 87% |
| Niacin (Vit $B_3$) | 32.9 mg | 164% | 30.8 mg | 154% |
| Vitamin $B_6$ | 3.8 mg | 191% | 1.9 mg | 96% |
| Folate* | 752 mcg | 188% | 492 mcg | 123% |
| Vitamin $B_{12}$ | 6.7 mcg | 112% | 3.0 mcg | 50% |
| Pantothenic acid (Vit $B_5$) | 8.9 mg | 89% | 2.7 mg | 27% |
| *Minerals* | | | | |
| Calcium | 614 mg | 61% | 834 mg | 83% |
| Iron | 21.2 mg | 118% | 19.2 mg | 107% |
| Magnesium | 496 mg | 124% | 258 mg | 64% |
| Phosphorus | 1,547 mg | 155% | 943 mg | 94% |
| Potassium | 5,205 mg | 149% | 2,319 mg | 66% |
| Sodium | 2,709 mg | 113% | 3,065 mg | 127% |
| Zinc | 14.1 mg | 94% | 9.3 mg | 62% |
| Copper | 2.3 mg | 114% | 1.0 mg | 51% |
| Manganese | 4.9 mg | 246% | 2.1 mg | 104% |
| Selenium | 134 mcg | 191% | 87.4 mcg | 125% |

*continues*

*continued*

| Nutrient | Paleo | %Calories | Western | %Calories |
|---|---|---|---|---|
| *Fatty Acid Profile* | | | | |
| Saturated | 28% | | 38% | |
| Monounsaturated | 45% | | 13% | |
| Polyunsaturated | 19% | | 18% | |
| Omega-3 | 4,700 mg | | 315 mg | |
| Omega-6 | 17,300 mg | | 10,678 mg | |
| Omega-6:Omega-3 (goal is 4:1 or lower) | 3.7:1 | | 34:1 | |
| Trans fat | 0 g | | 0 g | |

*Data prepared by* nutritiondata.com

*\*The folate that is found in the Western diet often comes in the form of folic acid in enriched refined grains. Folic acid is not easily utilized by the body and is not efficiently turned into folate, the nutrient our bodies actually need. Folic acid has actually been correlated with increased rates of certain cancers. The folate in the Paleolithic diet is from natural sources that are easily used by the body.*

# Key Points

Here are some key points to keep in mind when comparing the Paleolithic diet against the typical Western diet:

- **Calcium.** It's interesting to note that for every single vitamin and mineral value except for sodium, vitamin D, and calcium, the Paleolithic diet scores higher than the Western diet—sometimes by a landslide. For more information on why the calcium levels in the Paleolithic diet aren't alarming, see Chapter 2.

- **Cholesterol.** Despite the fact that we've been told over and over again that dietary cholesterol can lead to heart disease, the research just doesn't support that. For more information on why you shouldn't worry about the higher levels of cholesterol in this diet, read Chapter 4.

- **Vitamin D.** The vitamin D in the Western diet mostly comes in the form of the synthetic vitamin D used to fortify dairy. The best way to get vitamin D is through daily sun exposure, eating organ meats, and supplementation. We discuss supplementation and vitamin D more in Chapter 5.

- **Glycemic load.** The glycemic load score is a way of describing how much a particular food increases blood sugar. The Western diet has almost three times the effect on blood sugar as the Paleolithic diet.

- **Fatty acid profile.** It's interesting to note that the saturated fat content is lower and the monounsaturated fat (olive oil, animal foods) content is higher in the Paleolithic diet. One of the main arguments against the diet is that all the animal foods will contribute too much saturated fat. We discuss the fallacy that saturated fat causes heart disease in Chapter 4.

- **Omega-6 to omega-3 ratio.** What is likely one of the biggest causes of heart disease is the overload of omega-6s in the Western diet. One of the main goals of eating Paleo is to even out that astronomical omega-6 to omega-3 ratio. Judging by the scores in this category, Paleo seems to be doing just that.

# Index

## W-X-Y-Z